DATE

OPERATING ROOM CONFIDENTIAL

OPERATING ROOM CONFIDENTIAL
WHAT REALLY GOES ON WHEN YOU GO UNDER

by Paul Whang, MD

Published by ECW Press, 2120 Queen Street East, Suite 200
Toronto, Ontario, Canada M4E 1E2
416.694.3348 / info@ecwpress.com

LIBRARY AND ARCHIVES CATALOGUING IN PUBLICATION
Whang, Paul, 1956-
Operating room confidential :
what really goes on when you go under / Paul Whang.

ISBN 978-1-55022-918-9

1. Operating rooms—Popular works. I. Title.

RD31.5.W43 2010   617'.917   C2009-905962-2

Cover design: David Gee
Cover image: iStock Photo
Type: Melissa Kaita
Printing: Webcom   1   2   3   4   5

 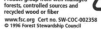 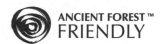

Mixed Sources
Product group from well-managed
forests, controlled sources and
recycled wood or fiber
www.fsc.org Cert no. SW-COC-002358
© 1996 Forest Stewardship Council

FSC

ANCIENT FOREST™
FRIENDLY

The publication of *Operating Room Confidential* has been generously supported by the
Canada Council for the Arts, which last year invested $20.1 million in writing and
publishing throughout Canada, by the Ontario Arts Council, by the Government of
Ontario through Ontario Book Publishing Tax Credit, by the OMDC Book Fund, an
initiative of the Ontario Media Development Corporation, and by the Government of
Canada through the Book Publishing Industry Development Program (BPIDP).

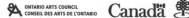 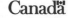

ONTARIO ARTS COUNCIL
CONSEIL DES ARTS DE L'ONTARIO   Canada   Canada Council   Conseil des Arts
                                                        for the Arts   du Canada

PRINTED AND BOUND IN CANADA

ECW PRESS
ecwpress.com

CONTENTS

To Susan, Matthew and Alexandra

INTRODUCTION

I am the person who calms and reassures you before the surgery begins and the last person you see before I gently transport you into unconsciousness. I watch over your body while the surgeon slashes and cuts, ensuring that your heart is protected from the stress and that oxygen is delivered to your vital organs. I keep you warm and give you blood if needed. Afterwards, I'll wake you up, making sure you don't throw up. I'm also the person who relieves your pain with numbing needles and I administer epidurals to women in labor. Yes, I'm your friendly hospital anesthetist.

I entered into this specialty because I like to work with others, both inside and outside of the operating room, and I can help patients to feel better as they heal — even after their bodies have been cut apart and stitched back together. Anesthesiology is about reducing pain, inducing amnesia or unconsciousness and putting a patient into a protected state of suspended animation during the stress of surgery.

I've always been fascinated by the physiology of the body and this is a common reason anesthetists enter this field — we want to understand the inner workings of important body organs. We learn to obsessively measure, manipulate, control and tinker with the body's function during an operation, using various devices and drugs. It sounds a bit nerdy — and it is. Only individuals with a certain personality would care about these things, and, as discussed in a later chapter about the characteristics of different specialists, anesthetists do share a particular personality and attention to detail.

We consider ourselves to be your advocate before your surgery even begins. We give the final okay that allows the surgery to proceed. If we think you aren't stabilized or won't survive the operation, we're not going to put you to sleep — it's just not going to happen.

Because we have this "permissive" role in the operating room, the relationship between surgeon and anesthetist is a curious one. Though there is a layer of professional courtesy and respect between the specialties, when either party scratches the surface, conflict can suddenly arise. Anesthetists are grateful that surgeons give us patients to anesthetise. But we curse when presented with patients who are missing important laboratory investigations or are ill prepared for the stresses of surgery. Surgeons, on the other hand, need us for the operation to happen in the first place, but they hate to be delayed or have the case canceled by us. However, like it or not, we both need each other. The frequent ribbing that occurs between us underscores the tension based upon this sometimes tense, yet symbiotic relationship.

Some people mistakenly assume that anesthetists receive assignments to work with particular surgeons for a day. In fact, I choose the operating room that I want to work in the day before. Obviously, monetary incentive plays a role for an anesthetist; the riskier and more difficult a case, the greater the starting fee charged, and the longer a surgery takes, the better it pays. Then there are occasions when I just want to be involved with a certain type of operation, like vascular or orthopedic surgery. But other considerations are also important. Working with a dull, humorless and cranky surgeon makes for a very long, boring day — and that's enough for me to switch rooms. On the other hand, working with a happy and engaged team makes the day fly by, and I finish work feeling good. Personal chemistry is so important; some people make me feel relaxed and at ease, while others rub me the wrong way. Let's face it — no matter what job you have, your satisfaction is influenced by those with whom you interact.

While caring for the patient in the operating room, I have a unique perspective — not that of the surgeon, assistant or nurse, who are all focused on the surgical field under the hot lights — but that of an observer, standing by the patient's sleeping face while his or her body is opened and dissected, noting the way others in the room react during the operation. I can observe the rhythms and routines of the operating room as the drama of surgery unfolds.

I decided to write this book for a number of reasons. First, people are curious about the operating room and hospital as is evident in the proliferation of fictional and documentary television shows and films set there. I was also motivated to expose the misconceptions many people have. After working in the O.R. for years, I now take for granted the routines and experiences of the operating room; it has become all so familiar. Yet, I recall my wide-eyed surprise and amazement when my own misunderstandings were first corrected. Thus, I can empathize with people's need for knowledge.

Another inspiration to write this occurred after reading Anthony Bourdain's wonderful book *Kitchen Confidential: Adventures in the Culinary Underbelly*. He revealed the behind-the-scenes, hidden world of cooking, chefs and restaurants — what really goes on behind the kitchen doors. The stories were a revelation to me. In the same way, I hope my book shines light on interesting aspects of hospital life for the uninitiated.

I also wanted to give some practical advice to those who have to come into hospital. Hospitals can be chaotic places, with strange antiseptic smells and confusing, endless corridors. They can be frightening. If you must come, you will probably be tested or probed by mysterious devices, possibly into some of your most private regions; you may have something scraped, cut out, sewn or fastened together while under sedation or a general anesthetic.

You will want to know how much pain you'll feel after the procedure. Are you going to feel nauseated? Are you going to be able to even pee without personal assistance or the use of a catheter?

You will also want to know something about the doctors

looking after you, such as the specific skills they bring to their jobs and what to expect from them.

I work all over the hospital — I'm in the labor and delivery room helping the obstetrician and easing labor pain. I'm in the diagnostic suites, where specialists like gastroenterologists and radiologists need sedation for patients undergoing procedures. I know which surgeon I'd want to operate on me — and which surgeon I would not allow to operate on my dog. I get to know the specialists and nurses who work outside of the operating room. Thus, I'm positioned at a hub in the hospital with a good finger on its pulse.

Though there are many interesting stories written or dramatized from the perspective of medical students learning to become doctors, there are not many day-to-day descriptions of life in the operating room and hospital. I want to illuminate these realities and share some of my personal feelings and experiences as an anesthetist in a busy community hospital.

The stories in the book are all based on real events and facts, derived from many different hospitals, and I guarantee you won't see me retracting fabrications on *Oprah*. That being said, many names of patients and doctors have been changed — to protect the innocent and, occasionally, to hide the guilty.

CHAPTER 1

A Day in the Operating Room

The operating room is the heart of the hospital where dramatic events and major, life-altering decisions occur. I'm sure that most people have no idea about some of the strange, unusual and unexpected events that occur here. You can watch shows like *ER, Grey's Anatomy* and *House* and think you know what's going on — but in fact you really don't.

I'm going to describe what working in the operating room is truly like. Hopefully, I can help you experience the operating room from a different perspective.

For many, a trip to the operating room is a frightening experience. You're going "under the knife," facing the unknown.

But I want to reassure you that you'll be cared for by an experienced team that is intimately acquainted with the routines and rhythms of the O.R. And though some team members may have unusual personalities and follow what may seem to be strange rituals, they have a lot of pride in their work and will care for you to the best of their abilities.

Every department in the hospital strives to attain the accepted "Standards of Care." In the O.R., the goals are not just to attain, but to exceed those standards — not only because we are directly responsible for people's lives, but also because it's what most of us demand from ourselves in our work. It may seem trite, but it is true — the operating room *is* the beating heart of the hospital.

Greens

Each day starts with the act of going into the locker room to change into surgical greens. Like a hockey player who puts his jersey and equipment on before a game, we prepare for a day in surgery by donning greens, slipping on the surgical cap and tying the mask.

O.R. greens are not designed for comfort or style. If you're not of average height or build, they definitely won't fit well. Their function is to keep you clean and relatively cool. There was a time, working as a resident at a downtown teaching hospital, when the greens weren't separate tops and bottoms, but were composed of a single jumpsuit. Male residents loved these jumpsuits, because they titillated us with the deep V that exposed the cleavage of female residents, who struggled to cover up. We couldn't fail to notice how tightly these suits hugged their bodies. Our eyes were very adept at outlining the braless attributes of certain classmates.

Instruments

A buzz of activity starts each morning, as the nurses in each room prepare for the day's surgeries. Pre-wrapped surgical instruments, specialized solutions and sheets of synthetic fibers that act as barriers to infection, called surgical drapes, are opened on sanitized stainless steel trays.

Because of the complexity of modern surgery and the myriad instruments used during each procedure, one is almost assured that some instrument will be missing or mistakenly substituted. This inevitably causes a delay in the proceedings. Curse-filled and panic-stricken calls from each operating room to SPD (Sterile Processing Department) ensure the proper instruments are sent up immediately.

I always find it curious that many surgical instruments are named after dead surgeons. Instead of "blunt-ended suction," it's called a *Yankauer*. In place of the "three-fingered clawed retractor," we use a *Senn-Miller*. I suppose it's an honor to have a surgical instrument that has saved many lives named after you, like a *Balfour Retractor* or *Allis Forceps*. And it's certainly easier to ask for the *Balfour Retractor* than the "adjustable self-retaining retractor with fenestrated side blades."

Despite the honor, there are certain instruments I'd rather not have my name associated with — I'm not sure how Dr. Pratt *really* felt about the *Pratt Rectal Speculum*.

However, I shouldn't make light of names. On a personal note, when I was beginning my anesthesia practice, I asked Dr. Robert Stubbs if I could work in his private cosmetic clinic. Dr. Stubbs is well known in the plastic surgery world as one of the first doctors who began penis enlargement surgery in North America.

"Wow, your name is Dr. Whang. Did you know that I learned the technique of penis enlargement in China with ... and I'm not kidding ... with Drs. Long and Dong. So you can just see my advertisement: *Penis enlargement surgery with Dr. Stubbs. Trained by Drs. Long and Dong. Anesthesia by Dr. Whang.*"

I didn't get the job.

Nurses

Operating room nurses are obviously a vital part of the O.R. team. There is currently an extreme shortage of qualified nurses in all areas of the hospital because there are an insufficient number of nurses coming up through the ranks — and this is especially evident in the O.R. Many of the most experienced nurses will be retiring within the next five to ten years. Some hospitals are filling these positions with nurses from other countries. One hospital is hiring nurses from the Philippines, while another hospital is employing many Russian nurses, yet another hospital is hiring Indian nurses and so on. In fact, most of us in North America should be feeling some guilt because we're depriving other countries of these caring and highly competent professionals.

I've observed two notable consequences of hiring foreign-trained healthcare workers at our hospitals. First, potluck lunch selections are now wonderful: succulent Ad Bong Baboy (chunks of pork cooked in soy sauce, vinegar, garlic, pepper and bay leaf) from the Philippines, wholesome Russian Lekeh (a honey pastry with raisins and walnuts) and tasty Indian Kalcha (bread made with flour, potatoes, onions, spices and butter).

Second, there is a new operating room vernacular — *specimen bottle* becomes *spacemen bootle*, *clamp* becomes *clemp*, and *room changeover* is now *room chenga over*. It's an adjustment for everyone.

The addition of nurses from different ethnic backgrounds has significantly changed the O.R. from its days of meat and potatoes and Queen's English. It has significantly spiced up both the lunchroom and the local vernacular.

Many people in North America don't consider a nursing career in the operating room appealing. First, some don't believe they can stand the blood and guts of operations — though in truth, only a small percentage of people *can't* tolerate it — and I have known a few who fainted observing their first operation and then went on to enjoy fulfilling operating room careers.

Some think that nursing in general doesn't pay well. The dearth of available nurses has emphasized their importance and recent contract agreements have significantly increased incomes.

The sway nurses have in the O.R. is changing every day. More nurses are training to become surgical assistants and fill manpower gaps in place of doctors. I've seen veteran nurses teach and advise doctors how to correctly set up and use new O.R. instruments since they often have more exposure and experience with the equipment than some surgeons.

The new rules instituting a safety checklist in the operating room, that must be followed before surgery can begin, reinforce the fundamental principle of teamwork, encourage us to look out for each other and stress the equal importance of every member in the team. In the past, I've seen warnings from experienced nurses prevent disaster. Unfortunately, advice ignored has resulted in some dangerously close calls. It's folly not to listen to an experienced voice in the O.R. In the old days, perhaps 30 to 40 years ago, doctors' treatment of nurses was sometimes abusive. At that time surgeons were considered to be the gods of the O.R. There were no policies to prevent and condemn bullying. There are legendary stories about doctors' raging tantrums and verbal tirades when things didn't go well. Doctors threw sponges and instruments, including scalpels, across the room . . . sometimes at others.

An older colleague recounted a good illustration of this behavior to me. A foul-mouthed bully of a surgeon was working with a veteran scrub nurse. During the surgery, he repeatedly demanded the wrong instruments from the nurse — for example, he'd ask for sutures when he wanted a scalpel. He blamed these errors on the nurse. "You should *know* what I need during the operation," he yelled. "How many times have *you* seen this operation? Give me what I *need*, not what I *ask for*!"

Finally, after being handed another "incorrect" scalpel, in self-righteous disgust he tossed it at her. She shifted back and it flew past her. Without hesitation, she immediately grabbed another scalpel from the instrument tray, cocked her wrist and deftly threw it at him — it whizzed just past his right eye, jangling onto the floor behind him. The O.R. was silent as the doctor stared at the nurse, his eyes wide with shock and fear. After this brief pause, the surgery resumed.

Little did he know that she was a competitive dart champion.

In the end, there were no complaints filed by either nurse

or surgeon; back then, things just weren't done that way. And neither uttered a word to each other about the incident.

But the surgeon never threw a surgical instrument at anyone again.

The Scrub

Nurses, surgeons and surgical assistants begin the scrub at the sinks just outside the O.R. "Scrubbing" is a ritual application of sterilizing soap solutions lasting at least five minutes, during which the definition of "clean" nails and hands achieves a standard that even Mom would appreciate. After finishing your scrub, you're not allowed to touch anything unsterile. Inevitably, the most exasperating itches seem to occur on the nose or eyes just after the hands are scrubbed, forcing people to beg others to scratch the offending area for them. If no one is available, you witness an odd sight — people desperately rubbing their faces against I.V. (intravenous) poles, tables or other sharp objects.

Surgically Clean

Of course, infection is the scourge of the O.R. Every attempt is made to prevent the introduction of bacteria, viruses and spores into or near surgical wounds. Sterility is an obsession.

"Surgically clean" means that even the slightest sneeze directed at the instruments, or even the simple suspicion of an unwashed hand grazing the corner of a surgical tray demands a replacement of the entire set. The touch of an unsterilized finger could deposit hundreds of thousands, if not millions, of microbes on an instrument, leading to a potentially life-threatening infection if deposited within the body.

And so, you can see there's definitely no adherence to the "five-second rule" for instruments that accidently fall to the floor.

For the germ-phobic obsessive-compulsive and other neurotic types of people who work in the operating room, these standards are perfect. It's as close to "Clean Nirvana" as it gets.

Waiting for the Call

Patients sit in the preoperative holding area, worrying and waiting to be called for surgery. Medical histories have been reviewed, with identification and allergy bands fastened to wrists. They shiver nervously under their flimsy gowns.

Many are surprised by how thin and revealing these gowns are. The old "Johnny gown" had the strings tied from behind leaving the back and buttock bare. Newer kimono-style gowns are better, but can still be revealing. Men who've never worn dresses are frequently guilty of exposing themselves. Large, hairy male patients sit oblivious, with legs spread wide apart, or ankle resting upon the opposite knee, groins uncovered, while seated opposite female patients who squirm uncomfortably, heads and bodies turned abruptly away to avoid seeing the genitalia on display. Believe me, it's happened on more than a few occasions.

People are given blankets to keep warm. Some wear them like shawls, loosely draped over shoulders. Others wrap them around their necks like scarves. There's even a small group that cover their heads, as if wanting to disappear and hide under cloaks. But many just leave the folded blankets unused upon their laps. These blankets should be used by the patient to keep as warm as possible. It's been shown that raising your temperature before surgery helps keep you warm during and after the operation. Even mild drops in temperature during and after an operation have been shown to significantly increase the risk of infection, blood loss or heart complications and prolong recovery room times.

The surgeon visits the patient just before surgery to mark the correct side with an "X" and answer any outstanding questions. After having already spent long detailed sessions in the office explaining the reasons for surgery, techniques and possible complications, there is sometimes a pained and exasperated look upon the surgeon's face when the patient asks: "Doc, tell me again — what are you going to do to me today?"

The Atmosphere

What about the tense atmosphere of the operating room among the nurses, surgeon and aneothctist? Between the sterility issues and the technical demands on the staff, you can often cut the tension in the air with a scalpel, so we definitely try to keep things loose and relaxed whenever possible. It's not always as serious as it's dramatized on TV shows — "Scalpel, please nurse! This cut determines whether the patient lives or dies!" In reality, no one could tolerate that kind of intensity with every operation, every day. We'd all go mad. Instead, the aim is to have a relaxed atmosphere and a day without complications. The conversation during operations ranges from sports scores and events in the news, to the latest O.R. and hospital gossip.

Some subjects come up repeatedly. We discuss recent difficult or unusual cases (while maintaining patient confidentiality): "He was barely hanging on — recent heart attack, pneumonia, kidney failure, massively obese — and the family still wanted everything done. When I suggested it looked hopeless and maybe we shouldn't do an operation, they threatened to kill me. I had to call security."

Foolish administrative decisions are regular joke fodder. These decisions usually concern manpower, equipment and how to save money, and we resent the fact that these decisions are made without consulting us, the ones directly affected by any changes. In a typical example, they once chose to switch to cheaper, inferior bandages — which ultimately resulted in increased costs, since we had to use twice as many bandages — but no one bothered to ask us our opinion.

Finally, we often discuss the recent behavior of quirky characters who work in the operating rooms — the ones we love, though they drive us nuts. Like the assistant who never stops releasing silent but deadly farts during surgery or another who endlessly complains about everything in the O.R; the orthopedic surgeon whose non-stop jabbering earned him the nickname Dr. BBC; the internist who appears only at night to see pre-op patients (that would be Dr. Vampire); the hyperactive, boyish, bouncy, obsessive-compulsive and talented ophthalmologist whom nurses want to strangle after hearing him say, "It went perfectly, perfectly fine" to every patient at the end of every operation, 15 times a day.

Music

Music helps the team relax and is a vital part of the preoperative routine. Each person has his or her favorite work soundtrack. Whether it's hard rock or classical music, it's amusing to see how important music is to some people, particularly surgeons. Some surgeons will even refuse to start surgery unless their radio station or personal CD is playing. Some will refuse to start if there is rap music playing. Personally, I don't like country music for the operating room — there's already going to be a lot of hurtin' going on. One surgeon I work with will not sew up the surgical wound unless a particular piece is playing. On many occasions, the operating room staff votes to select a certain style that everyone enjoys.

Sometimes the choice of music can create some funny situations — like the time "Hurts So Good" was playing just before a hip replacement, or when "Stairway to Heaven" played before I put a patient to sleep.

O.R. Voodoo

Another strange preoperative ritual is "O.R. Voodoo." Like athletes who have specific pre- or post-game rituals, such as always eating steak or tying their shoes the same way, many doctors have routines they religiously follow before or during the operation. One surgeon drives along the same route to the hospital every day, regardless of the weather or traffic conditions. Another surgeon, when closing a wound, will count every suture she makes — and if she ends on 13, she will either take one suture out or add an extra one to make it "right." Some feel they must sterilize the skin in a certain manner before the operation can even begin.

The majority of operations go smoothly and completely as planned. However, in the back of our minds, based on our collective experience, we all know this can change. The tone of the O.R. can quickly go from calm at one moment to disaster in an instant. All it takes is a sudden anaphylactic allergic reaction, a laceration of a major artery, an accidental cut to a major nerve or organ . . . the list goes on. O.R. Voodoo creates the magic spell warding off the bad luck lurking in the shadows. Hell, if it would help me avoid a bad outcome, I'd go to the O.R. nude.

The Bad Karma of VIPs

Even before surgery begins, you might wonder if there are factors that increase your risk of complications. Are there circumstances that create negative karmic energy during your operation, leading to a bad outcome? Most definitely, the answer is yes. This occurs especially when the patient is a doctor, lawyer, nurse, hospital volunteer or even just the spouse of one of these individuals. If any of the staff comments during the operation that "Everything is going so smoothly" or "We'll be going home soon" — get ready for trouble.

If one or any combination of these factors applies to you before surgery, be very, very afraid. Here are just a few examples of problems that have arisen in these situations: a transplanted knee ligament unexpectedly falls from the surgeon's hand onto the cold and unsterile floor (doctor's wife); partial paralysis occurs after an epidural insertion (nurse); the main blood vessel to the gut is accidentally cut, instead of the kidney vessel (lawyer's mother); unexplained fluctuations in the blood pressure and pulse occur during a major hip operation requiring intensive care admission (hospital volunteer).

I don't know why there seems to be increased risk with patients who are or are associated with lawyers, nurses, hospital volunteers or doctors, but believe me, there definitely is. Maybe the extra pressure causes the operating room staff to change their normal routines and thus make mistakes. As Voltaire said, "The enemy of good is perfect." Just knowing that you're operating on a high-risk patient causes you to second-guess every move: how a surgeon would normally approach incisions and suturing might change or an anesthetist might decide to modify doses and add or subtract new drugs. Everyone must constantly fight the urge to make it "just a little bit better" for the VIP. I've noticed that my hands develop a small, disconcerting tremor under such circumstances. In fact, for me, the entire mood in the operating room changes. The music disappears, the surgeon doesn't chatter, assistants refrain from commentary, nurses stop gossiping and time slows.

Inadvertently commenting that things are going smoothly during an operation curses everyone. This is self-explanatory — the O.R. Gods punish those who arrogantly believe that mere mortals control their own destiny. If, during an operation, any fool dares to make such a statement, they are immediately shouted down and rebuked by the rest of us.

Assistants

Most surgeons work with a surgical assistant, especially during larger operations. In my experience, the majority of assistants are very good. Good assistants anticipate the surgeon's every move, retracting and suctioning blood to expose and clear the operative site. There is an old but true surgical axiom — the key to good surgery is "exposure, exposure, exposure."

On the other hand, a poor assistant can make a surgeon's life hell. Many times I've heard the sickening thud and witnessed the subsequent minor contusion suffered by the surgeon, caused by an inadvertent head-butt by the assistant. I've seen the phenomenon of "assistant eclipse," as the assistant's head slowly blocks illumination from the overhead operating room lights, casting an ominous shadow over the operative site. Finally, there is the dreaded "cut wrong thing," as in, cut the wrong suture, or cut the surgeon's finger (when this happens we say the assistant is guilty of "surgeonocide").

There are also assistants who — how can I put it? — are a bit odd. Some endlessly babble on about their personal struggles, holding the rest of us captive during an operation. Many use the operating room as a personal psychotherapy session. With one assistant, we have had to endure the story of his marital breakup, divorce, verbal battles with his ex-spouse and adventures with online dating. Another drones on about her shortcomings and weight gain, outlining what fat does to her hips. There seems to be no detail too embarrassing or intimate to discuss in the O.R. We all grimly work on in uncomfortable silence, hoping that our lack of interest will discourage them — it never does.

Of course, the surgeon needs the assistant and thus forges on, teeth clenched painfully behind his or her mask.

Finally, we have the "old veteran" assistant. Like a player past his prime, it's difficult to tell him it's time to quit. One older assistant has angina and diabetes and has had a heart bypass and knee replacement surgery. He's fainted during operations at least three times — fortunately not fainting *into* the patient. After each episode, the whole gamut of neurological and cardiac tests was performed with no definitive answers. It is obvious to us that he's getting a bit old, and the job is too stressful for him. Many have thought that he should let go of the retractor and enjoy life. Though he's been stable for the last few months, it's disconcerting to have to watch over the assistant as well as the patient.

The Cold Operating Rooms

Once all the preparation is done, the patient enters the operating room. What's surprising to most people is how bone-chillingly cold it is — it's as if someone forgot to pay the gas bill. Of course, patients are forced to wear those utterly embarrassing, unappealing, thin operating room gowns — the "Johnny gowns" that tie and open in the back, displaying your ass for the world to see. (Newer gowns have recently been developed that better preserve one's dignity, but they're not commonly used yet.) It's as if the hospital decided to find the least warm, most humiliating piece of clothing for patients to wear in one of the coldest rooms in the building.

Operating rooms are intentionally kept cool. Around the operating table, the staff is wearing thick waterproof surgical gowns, at least two layers of thick gloves and surgical caps. On top of that, they're standing under intense, bright and very hot surgical lights. Unless you want a surgeon, nurse and assistant to collapse with heat exhaustion, just accept the fact it's got to be cool.

What Not to Say Just Before Your Surgery

I must warn you that before the operation starts, there are two things you should never say to the operating room staff.

First, please try to avoid saying, "If you guys don't do a good job, I'm going to sue you all." This tends to cause the tension in the room to rise and any feelings of goodwill that existed will rapidly dwindle. The operating team has a lot of pride in our jobs and we work to the best of our abilities. We do not need to be threatened or coerced into doing a better job — it's an insult. None of us need to be preoccupied with the threat of a potential lawsuit. We're trying to take care of you.

Second, when you're asked repeatedly about your medical history, drug allergies or to confirm the side of the operation, try not to joke or playfully mislead anyone. It may seem like the tenth time you've been asked the same thing, but safety and your wellbeing are our primary concern. That's why making a crack about which side of your body is going under the knife is akin to joking about a bomb to airport security — no one's going to laugh. We are all familiar with hospital horror stories about a patient having the wrong leg amputated. At one hospital where I worked, the surgeon removed the healthy lung of a smoker, tragically leaving the patient to die with his remaining cancer-filled lung.

These mistakes happen for many reasons. It can be as simple as the surgeon not checking the x-ray notes to confirm the correct side. There can be a language barrier that goes undetected or a communication problem no one bothers to clarify. Even after the surgeon checks the side, the assistant and nurses in the operating room may clean and drape the wrong side before the surgery starts. The surgeon, entering the room, may assume that all the usual preoperative checks had been performed and begin the surgery.

It amazes me how many patients are in an almost disassociated state before their operations. They don't speak up when things are obviously incorrect. They answer yes to all questions, passively following instructions. We've been socialized into handing over our care and security to medical personnel and somehow give up our responsibility at the doors of the operating room.

I have witnessed an eerie occurrence where two patients, roughly the same age, both named Smith, were mixed up — one was to have a cataract operation, while the other was to have a circumcision. The wrong Mr. Smith was called by the nurse to accompany him to the operating room.

Needless to say, there was great relief when the mistake was found just before Mr. Smith's eye was draped, ready to be cut. We can only imagine the shock and surprise of the second Mr. Smith, had the other operation been carried out.

So please don't joke about which side or what part is to be operated upon. It amplifies the paranoia that we already have.

Starting the Intravenous

Now we've prepared for the operating room, the staff is ready and you enter the chilly room in your flimsy gown. After lying on the operating table, an anesthetist will start the intravenous. Many patients say this is "the scariest part of the procedure."

This is a pet peeve of mine. Let's get real, people. The anesthetist is going to stick a small needle, slightly bigger than the size of a sewing needle, into your vein. Contrast this with what the surgeon is about to do. He is going to make a large cut through your skin and cause you to bleed. Then he'll stretch, scrape, clamp and cut another part of your body. Yet my small intravenous is "the worst part of the operation." Let's give the anesthetist a break and tell your surgeon to be careful.

Paradoxically, other than small children — whom everyone understandably sympathizes with — some of the most terrified patients are large, muscular men with numerous tattoos depicting evil, death and destruction covering their arms, chest and back. These are men who have already endured thousands of un-anesthetized needles! I still can't get over the look of terror — panic-filled eyes, cold sweaty foreheads and trembling arms — as I approach them with my needle.

For some, the needle may conjure up some childhood experience that scarred them for life. And the patient might see the needle as a symbol for the surgery that is to follow. But to me, when all is said and done, it's still just a little needle.

Reactions Just Before Sleep

Most patients justifiably feel some apprehension right before the anesthetic is given. I've noticed different kinds of reactions prior to unconsciousness.

First are the Type A personalities, many of them businessmen. It's the idea of losing control, more than the risk of complications, that terrifies them the most. They hide this fear with a blank mask while on the operating table. Responses to questions are monosyllabic grunts — yes or no. Blood pressures zoom sky-high and heart rates gallop into the mid-hundreds.

It's easy to quantify anxiety by measuring the vital signs. Calming words of reassurance tend not to help. It's best to get these people to sleep pronto.

The second group are those who indulge in recreational drugs. The narcotics given just before going to sleep are, for them, an enjoyable, familiar and free high. Like the dreadlocked Rastafarian, who, after being injected with morphine really did exclaim, "That good ganja, give me more that shit!" Or the patient whose nose was filled with cocaine-soaked cotton balls (to contract blood vessels and reduce bleeding, prior to starting nasal surgery), whose eyes popped wide open with excitement as he asked, "That's cocaine, isn't it? Tell me!"

But the big problem with drug users is their incredible resistance to the anesthetic drugs. Their bodies develop a tremendous tolerance. Giving double doses of sleep medicines often only results in a confused stare and the question — "Hey man, when am I going to sleep?" You've got to bring out the really big syringes for these people.

Propofol

The most common drug used to put you to sleep is propofol. Because the drug is suspended in a milky white emulsification derived from soybean oil, some people call it "milk of amnesia." The drug itself causes many to experience a painful burning sensation when it's injected, so it's often mixed with some local anesthetics. Introduced many years ago, it has tremendous advantages over the old standby, sodium thiopental. Propofol quickly puts patients to sleep after injection (it takes the drug 20 to 30 seconds to reach the brain after it's injected), and it rapidly washes out of the brain when regaining consciousness. Once awake, most people become clear-headed very quickly, with significantly less nausea than with sodium thiopental. It can also be used as a continuous infusion to keep people unconscious for many hours.

The dangers of propofol have recently been highlighted with the death of Michael Jackson. It can cause breathing to slow or even stop and drops the blood pressure. There is tremendous variability in response, depending on age, disease and concomitant drug use. For example, in some frail elderly patients, I'll sometimes give one-sixth the dose I'd give to young adults, to avoid triggering a cardiac arrest. Experience with the drug and the ability to deliver oxygen into the lungs are absolute requirements before it can be used by an anesthetist.

Propofol has an interesting history. When it first came out, there were lots of rumors circulating about the erotic dreams that people recalled when they awoke. There were anecdotal stories about people waking up, saying that they had the most stimulating and wonderful dreams ever. In truth, most of this was the power of suggestion. Once people realized that it was just an expectation implanted in their minds, the stories decreased significantly.

It was indeed an interesting process. If you looked like Brad Pitt when giving an anesthetic, women would experience wild dreams. The same holds true for female anesthetists who looked like Halle Berry — the male patient would report having had fantastic dreams. To my disappointment, the only dreams my patients seem to remember are of going to the office or doing housework. For some reason, I inspire a lot of dreams about vacuuming.

Sensitivity to Anesthetic

What about sensitivity to anesthetics? Are there large differences in reactions to the drugs depending on your race or lifestyle? Yes.

If a patient is Asian, the dose of pain medicines and narcotics has to be generally reduced by 25 to 50 percent because of increased sensitivity. It's not unusual to have Asian patients wake up very slowly and remain drowsy hours after the operation — the "Oriental coma," as some recovery nurses call it. Asians also report a higher incidence of nausea and vomiting afterwards, especially women.

On the other hand, for elderly East Indian patients, the clearance and metabolism of drugs is amazingly fast. Even tiny, wizened Indian grannies will pop their eyes open at the end of an operation and ask for more pain medicine.

If you're a Brit who smokes and drinks, we know what to expect. In general, the dose of pain medicines and anesthetics needed is substantially larger than normal and you will wake up from an anesthetic very quickly. (As my English medical professor would proudly say to me in the pub, as he puffed on his cigarette and took another sip of Guinness, "We Brits can really handle drugs. Just look at Keith Richards.")

Smoking has some benefits with respect to anesthetics. Smokers have a significantly reduced incidence of nausea after anesthetics. However, the effects of smoking on the lungs and the heart tend to outweigh this sole benefit.

Surgery

Once the anesthetic has taken effect, the surgery can now begin. The area to be operated on is slathered and cleaned with copious amounts of sterilizing solutions at least twice. Drapes are then applied around the area of the skin to be cut. It is the moment of truth. The initial cut by the surgeon always causes the heart rate and blood pressure to rise in the sleeping patient as the body reacts to the pain in a reflexive, unconscious way. If the patient is not adequately paralyzed, the arms or legs may even jerk in response.

Occasionally, like a scene out of *The Twilight Zone*, the patient's hands will break free of the restraints and instinctively reach and grab at the area being operated on. Sometimes, the patient's right hand will inadvertently grab at the surgeon's butt through the sterile drapes. I find this has a tendency to irritate the surgeon.

During "open" (not keyhole) abdominal surgery, where a large cut exposes the gut, if there is inadequate muscle paralysis, muscles will tighten and push the writhing, squirming coils of pink guts through the cut and over the body, like coiled toothpaste squeezed from a tube. It's a very freaky but totally involuntary reflex.

As the surgeon cuts and probes deeper, the sleeping body tries to protect itself from this unnatural invasion and reactions become more and more intense. The anesthetic now needs to be "deepened" to blunt these responses.

The Quality of Your Tissue

Does the surgeon always judge the quality of the tissue operated upon, detecting differences in tissue strength and elasticity, as it is cut, drilled and sutured? Most definitely. During an operation, the surgeon will ascertain if the patient's tissue is firm and strong or weak and flabby. Some people are born with tough and robust tissue. Even the simple feel of the knife as it cuts through tissue or a suture as it pierces an organ indicates tissue strength. In other people, as a result of genetics or disease, the surgeon questions the strength of his repair due to the tissues. Surgeons frequently refer to this as "poor protoplasm."

In the end, doctors can easily determine your inner physical qualities and strengths, as they gauge drug reactions and peer into your body as easily as other people judge your external appearance and personality.

Electrocautery
Many people think that most surgery is carried out with sharp scalpels and knife-like cutting instruments. In fact, a lot of surgery — especially keyhole surgery which uses long, pincer-and-grabber instruments introduced through the body wall and viewed on cameras — is done with electrocautery currents. One hand holds and pulls the tissues with a pincer-like instrument, and the other hand burns and cuts tissue with an electrocautery probe. Like a *Star Wars* lightsaber, the sparking cautery tip melts tissue, accompanied by distinctive buzzing sounds and puffs of smoke.

The hazy, white smoke produced from burned tissue smells like a barbecue. Recently, serious concerns have been raised about secondhand smoke escaping into the operating room and the possible cancer risks. Also, disease-transmitting viruses may accompany the drifting smoke as infected tissue is burned. Because of these possible dangers, most electrocautery is combined with suction tubing. As the electrocautery occurs, smoke particles are sucked through nearby tubing and removed from the operating room. With the improved safety of the smoke evacuator, most of us don't mind giving up the smell of summer grilling.

We've come a long way since Dr. W. Bovie first used electrocautery in the operating room to cauterize bleeding vessels in 1906. Surgeons can work with metallic instruments flowing with electric currents, without feeling the jolts themselves. The surgical gloves offer protection by insulating them from the electric current.

Occasionally however, without warning, a microscopic hole can appear in the surgeon's glove. With the next press of the cautery button, a surgeon will yell in terrible pain and throw the cautery tool down. A very painful burn will be seen on the finger, in the area of the small hole. It's a hazard when working with electricity. It's one reason many surgeons, nurses and assistants double glove.

The risks of the electrocautery aren't limited to burning the surgeon. It can ignite fires within the patient as well.

There are documented cases of patients blowing up with the flammable gases — methane, produced by bacteria in the gut, and hydrogen, made by the fermentation and metabolism of digested carbohydrates. Surgeons have observed a flash accompanied by a bang and suffered facial burns with singed eyelashes and eyebrows. Some places in the intestines contain up to 40 percent flammable gases. Gallbladder surgery and operations of the intestines and stomach have been associated with explosions. It's not a common occurrence, but it's definitely quite memorable when it happens.

In our hospital, a patient having a colonoscopy to remove a polyp (small growth) had an explosion in his gut. There was a flash and a bang, and the patient's body nearly lifted off the bed. An entire section of intestine was torn, and had to be removed during emergency surgery. Fortunately, he survived.

The Untold Dangers of Sitting Down

We've discussed hazards, like explosive gases, intrinsically produced by the body. But the long list of items that people put *into* their bodies is another story.

Some humans feel the urge to insert objects into their rectum. This may be a regression to the anal retentive, sub-stage of psychosexual development, as hypothesized by Freud — on the other hand, they may just like the recreational fun and enjoyment of inserting things up their rectum. Unfortunately, a few of these objects will become lodged in the gut and have to be extracted under a general anesthetic. What many of these patients don't realize is that, like the promise of many pest-control traps, what goes in doesn't necessarily come out.

Because of the segmented, curved nature of the intestines, or the awkward edges of objects, things inserted into the long, winding intestines through the rectum can be very difficult to take out again.

The list of items we've seen inserted into the rectum includes fruits and vegetables, like bananas, cucumbers, squash and zucchini; all manner of balls, from tennis to billiard; shampoo, detergent and perfume bottles; and, as a sign of the modern age we live in, more and more vibrators.

Now, just a note: there are sex toys specifically made for anal use — just a reminder that serious complications can result unless form and function go hand in hand with appropriate use.

A colleague described an interesting vibrator extraction to me. After the patient was asleep, the surgeon identified the vibrator with its accompanying wires, by using a proctoscope (a lighted, long viewing scope that's inserted into the rectum). Numerous attempts to extract the vibrator were unsuccessful. Finally, with the use of long, pincer-like instruments, normally used for laparoscopic surgery, he was able to slowly pull it out.

It was the sudden, unexpected activation of the vibrator, while placed upon a metal tray, with its buzzing and rattling, that shocked and surprised everyone in the operating room. All were impressed by how the product obviously exceeded the minimum durability standards as read in the "excessive wear and tear" section of its warranty.

When asked how these objects came to be inserted into the rectum, most explanations are, of course, related to sexual activity. The other excuses — like "I just wanted to see what would happen when I did this" — cause many of us to scratch our heads in disbelief.

Our usual tact, delicacy and understanding are sorely (and too often) tested when the excuse "I accidentally sat on it" is used, especially in circumstances similar to the case of a gentleman who had a potato the size of a large grapefruit impacted in his rectum. You're probably not too surprised that many of us in the operating room had a difficult time imagining this to be an accident.

Our response in circumstances like these is usually, "Yeah, really? *Sure.*"

The objects inserted into the penis are obviously smaller (we hope) than those stuck up the rectum. These are usually chains, Q-tips and other long thin items. The most interesting case we've seen recently was a gentleman who had stereo wires tangled and caught into his penis. We assumed that he wanted to be wired for action *and* sound. These wires were successfully extracted after a cystoscopy (using a lighted scope inserted into the penis). We were all happy for the patient and for the fact that his stereo speakers could probably be used again.

Awareness During an Operation

What about "awareness" during an operation? We've all heard the horror stories of people claiming to be awake yet paralyzed while the surgeon is cutting and yanking at organs. The person wants to scream for help but can't. No one is aware that they're experiencing this nightmare. This definitely happens.

I know of a patient who complained that she was able to hear an entire conversation during gallbladder surgery. She recalled almost word for word the conversation between the anesthetist and the nurse about color preferences for a newly renovated kitchen. The patient tried to scream but couldn't because she was paralyzed. She recalled feeling the cold burning sensation of the knife as it slit the skin of her abdomen. The next thing that she remembered was the voice of the anesthetist saying, "Gee, her blood pressure and heart rate are kind of high. I better give her some anesthetic." Thankfully, the patient's nightmare ended and she lapsed into unconsciousness.

Awareness during surgery may occur as often as one to six out of a thousand cases. But I have to be honest — aside from unstable patients who can only tolerate minimal anesthetic or during Caesarean sections, where limited anesthetic is given to protect the baby — I believe that a lot of the awareness during routine operations is a result of anesthesia neglect: the failure to maintain adequate levels of drugs during the operation to keep the person asleep.

I've walked into operations where the anesthetist didn't notice that the vaporizer containing the anesthetic gases had run out. I've had to gently remind him — "Um ... I think you've run out of gas."

What follows is the shock of realization, then a desperate fumbling with the canister to refill the vaporizer and deepen the anesthetic. Sometimes drugs are given to induce amnesia, just in case awareness is occurring.

When this fact was revealed to a former newspaper editor, his first response was "Yikes!" He thought this revelation about drugs to induce amnesia was a trick to avoid a lawsuit. In fact, he's correct. With the injection of the amnesic drug, any memories of awareness would hopefully be wiped out and ongoing awareness stopped — and a potential lawsuit avoided.

As I have written in my chapter, "The Good, the Bad and the Ugly" — which discusses doctor training and competency — doctors are not infallible and will make mistakes. This is the reality of medicine and life.

The best doctors recognize when mistakes occur and know how to quickly and competently correct the error so that the patient is not harmed.

When a patient experiences awareness, the anesthetist may have been preoccupied doing other tasks. (Tell your surgeon not to distract your anesthetist with a good joke at critical moments.) Some older anesthetic machines don't have warning alarms to tell you you're running low. Fortunately, no one has ever reported awareness during one of my anesthetics. But my colleagues and I have all experienced occasions where these potential problems have quickly been averted.

Connect accidental neglect with the fact that certain people are more resistant to the awareness blocking effects of anesthetic drugs and you have the potential for intraoperative awareness.

It may sound scary, but the anesthetist will aim to ensure that intraoperative awareness will not occur. There are brain monitors that can measure levels of awareness. In the end, though, it's really only the vigilance of the anesthetist that guarantees that you won't be listening to a surgical conversation or bad music during the operation.

The Missing Sponge

Before the patient can leave the operating room and before the operation is considered to be complete, the closing count of all instruments, sutures and sponges tallied at the beginning of surgery must equal the count at the end of surgery. Of course, leaving things in the body can be disastrous. For the patient it can mean chronic infections and can sometimes be life-threatening. For the physicians and nurses it can mean a potential lawsuit.

If the final count is wrong, a good day can quickly change into a bad day. A muffled groan erupts from the entire operating room team and signifies the start of a desperate search. The surgical field and drapes around the operative site are closely inspected. The gowns, hands and bodies of anyone beside the O.R. table are carefully scrutinized. Shoes, especially the soles, are examined. The perimeter as far as five to ten feet away from the operative site is searched. It's surprising how far small needles can fly or be carried on the soles of shoes to the other side of the room during an operation. Many of these are the size of nail clippings. Other times, things inadvertently become attached to the surgeon's gloves, arms and, in one memorable moment, to the surgeon's butt.

If you were to enter the operating room at this time, you would witness a very odd sight, like a Kafkaesque piece of performance art. You would see a silent group of people staring intently at the floor, looking lost and bewildered — some wandering like zombies, unblinkingly scanning the floor while others are on all fours, crawling around the operating table with faces just inches from the ground. All the while, the flashing lights and beeps of the anesthetic machine watch over the unconscious patient.

If by chance some eagle-eyed person finds the missing needle, there is a triumphant shout of "Found it!" followed by smiles, congratulations and high-fives.

I can personally say that on those rare occasions when I've found the missing object, I feel a goofy sense of pride. I feel as if I've won the door prize at a convention.

What happens if the needle or lost object can't be is found? A sense of gloom hangs over everyone. An x-ray must be taken of the entire body and is read by either the surgeon or a radiologist, in order to locate the missing object. This procedure can add another 20 or 30 minutes to the operating time. If the object is found in the body, it means re-exploration of the surgical site.

This can also be terribly frustrating. Think of trying to find objects like a tiny needle or a blood-soaked sponge the size of a small mothball in a body cavity filled with an overlapping, floppy mixture of organs and slippery tissue layers. It's the ultimate needle in a blood-filled haystack. It's a nightmare. Like I said, a good day becomes a very bad day.

Operating Room Sex

Because people work as a close-knit team under occasionally stressful conditions and in close proximity to each other, another question that is frequently asked concerns operating room romances and affairs. The answer is: it depends on the circumstances.

In the teaching hospitals, the incidence of operating-room sex is probably higher than in most community hospitals. Medical residents want to know about everything that goes on in the hospital, even sex. I remember there was screwing around among residents and hospital staff. The heady mix of youth, high hormone levels and tension created many amorous opportunities.

Certain trainees wanted to achieve some sexual goals before finishing their residency, such as doing it on the operating table.

This is not as awkward as one might think, since an O.R. table is a unique piece of apparatus that can be contorted into almost any sexually advantageous position that one would desire. At one hospital, the cleaning lady surprised the senior surgical resident testing the O.R. table in this way, as he pumped vigorously into an operating room nurse, whose legs were perfectly positioned in the stirrups of the operating table — the so-called lithotomy horny position. The cleaning lady fled screaming from the room. In another often-recounted episode, the chief of surgery was discovered enjoying a midday tryst on his office desk with an attractive surgical resident. Finally, a colleague told me she managed to sneak her boyfriend into the hospital on her last day of the rotation in order to fulfill her goal of doing it in the on-call room.

At other hospitals, a celibate monk would feel right at home. I believe the stress levels experienced by staff play a large part in determining the level of extra-curricular activity. However, it's not easy to predict and one can't always tell "who's doing who." To illustrate this point, let me tell the story of "Sukie" who was, until recently, on the staff of our hospital. She reminded me of a child's doll: she had a pale, almost white, small face framed by long, dark hair. She was barely five feet tall and weighed about 90 pounds. She would look away from you when greeted with "Good morning" and barely squeak an audible "Hello" in reply. She seemed to have the personality of a mouse.

After about six months, she moved to a nearby trauma and teaching hospital. This hospital accepts the most serious accidents of the region and is known to have a very stressful and high-energy work environment. Subsequent information from the grapevine indicated that Sukie had turned into a sexual vixen; she had screwed at least two staff people and two residents, one of whom had proposed marriage.

Teamwork

I've just discussed an intimate form of teamwork. The other kind of teamwork is the most important factor in determining good versus bad operating rooms. Despite the stress and the long hours, a strong sense of camaraderie and teamwork is key in motivating people to do a good job. There are several perks to compensate for this; however there is one important one. In the hospital, there is an unwritten rule that states if you are part of a hospital and team, you get to go to the front of the line, when you need to, even if the waiting list is six months long.

If you are a member of the O.R. team and need to see a doctor, the question becomes: "Are you available for an appointment this afternoon?" Got a sore shoulder? Dr. Smith, the orthopedic surgeon on call, will see you between cases, although he has an office full of people. And, if he determines that an operation is needed, he will make room on his O.R. list to have you done in two days.

Yes, this is queue jumping. And absolutely no one is going to stop us. As we say, there are few perks we receive during our job, but this is the one thing we can do to help each other out. Do tellers in their own bank wait in line to do their own transactions? Do vacationing pilots wait in a check-in line to fly their own airline? Obviously not. Queue jumping will occur whenever it will not endanger another life.

This story further illustrates the concepts and benefits of teamwork: one of our nurses was sideswiped on the highway. It was quite a serious accident, but she came into our emergency room still conscious, badly bruised on her left side but still talking. Word of her accident quickly spread to the operating room. She was thought to be stable, and one of the anesthetists went down to see her. Suddenly, she complained about shortness of breath and felt weak. She started to turn blue and lost consciousness. He desperately inserted a breathing tube into her airway, started some large fluid intravenous lines and called the operating room STAT (immediately). In the operating room, they diagnosed her as having a collapsed lung and ruptured spleen. Essentially, she couldn't breathe and had massive internal bleeding.

After the initial shock of her sudden collapse, the O.R. team flew into action. It was a hive of activity: three surgeons and three anesthetists worked feverishly to stabilize her and repair the damage. Other doctors strode in and asked to help. Any free nurse brought necessary instruments and blood into the operating room. Fortunately, she recovered, but the normal daily activity of the operating room ground to a halt. During this time, many patients waiting in the presurgical area, dressed in gowns, asked what was going on. An elderly lady — who had probably been waiting for months to have her knee done — limped up to the O.R. clerk and asked if the rumors were true and that we were operating on one of our nurses. When she was told we were, she said, "That's okay; tell them to take their time. All of us want her to be all right." Everybody knows we all have to help each other out, at one time or another.

CHAPTER 2

On Call in the House of Scream

The Pager

It's Friday and unfortunately, I'm on call. Over the next 24 hours, I'll be sleep deprived. Patients will be transferred from the emergency department to the operating room, where everything — from broken bones and infected gall bladders to ruptured aneurysms — will be mended, removed or repaired. The labor and delivery floor will call me for Caesarean sections and epidurals. In fact, any place in the hospital, from the emergency room to the patient wards, can call on me if someone has a cardiac arrest. Just thinking about all these medical emergencies makes me feel tired.

And even if I do have the opportunity to sleep, it's a restless, agitated sleep — expectantly waiting for my pager to ring. I don't know what they'll call me for or why they'll need me, but I have to be ready. The unexpectedness and randomness of the events adds to my stress. I'll wake up frequently, suspicious of a pager malfunction, a missed call or that I'm sleeping too well. It's a sad state to be in. When it is quiet and peaceful, I'm distressed by the serenity and become on edge again.

In fact, the pager becomes an accursed thing, the messenger that badgers and startles when you don't want to be disturbed — when you are sitting on the toilet, occupied with an important clinical task or just as your head snuggles into the soft pillow in anticipation of some blissful shut-eye.

After the seventh page in 20 minutes, I curse the pager as if it were a malicious living creature waiting to taunt me at every opportunity. I feel like smashing it against the wall. I know my Freudian subconscious is truly at work given the number of times the pager has fallen into the toilet — believe me, it can't be entirely accidental. But here's the sad thing: after drying it off, the damn thing still works, and the evil creature lives on.

Some hospitals have replaced pagers with cell phones. Even though cell phones may cost more, and there are dead zones where cell phones don't function, I've got to admit, I prefer the pager. Once a pager has stopped ringing, I can look at the display and then decide whether I want to respond to it right away. A ringing cell phone insists that I answer it and be connected with someone immediately. The pager offers me a choice.

I confess that when my pager indicates calls are coming from certain, noncritical wards, I'll wait for them to page me a second time before responding to give myself a little extra rest. After all, the wards have often confused me with Dr. Wang, a family doctor; Dr. Wong, an obstetrician; and Dr. Leong, a gastroenterologist. Don't we all look the same and have similar names? At least, that's my excuse.

My response to the pages deteriorates as the day progresses. Fatigue and irritation start to take their toll.

In the morning, it's "Hello. How are you? What can I do for you?"

By afternoon, it's "Anesthesia on call. What's the problem?"

By late evening, it's "Yeah? What is it?"

As I grow older, I prepare for being on call with increasing dread. I laugh at myself now, recalling that years ago, when I first started practice, I found being on call exciting. It presented an opportunity to apply my skills and knowledge, crystallized through years of study, to treat patients and overcome the challenges presented. It was like an adventure. Unfortunately, most of that excitement has been worn away and replaced with the burden of heavy responsibility and fatigue. Hopefully, I can always retain the sense that I am doing some good for others.

When I'm on call, especially late at night, I'm called to various patient wards in the hospital and each has its own distinct atmosphere and feel. When entering the softly illuminated patient wards at night, my footsteps echo down the darkened corridors. Sometimes, it feels like I'm entering the sanctuary of a monastery. It's a subdued atmosphere, where every effort is made to give peace and quiet to the patients — patients who have had to endure endless rounds of tests and procedures during the day and who are now seeking the solace and serenity of the night. When arriving at the nursing desk late at night, we try to preserve this peace and calm and speak in soft whispers.

In contrast, if you're called to the emergency room in a large urban hospital, it's truly like an episode of the television show *ER* — loud and chaotic, with paramedics constantly arriving with the injured and sick. Seriously ill patients are hustled to resuscitation rooms. The less seriously ill sit endlessly in the overcrowded waiting room, hoping to be next in line to see the emergency room doctor. The stress level on the nurses and doctors is very high. With some people, tension boils just below the surface.

Camaraderie is more difficult to foster in this environment. For example, if I ask, "Could you tell me where the order forms are?" an E.R. nurse might respond, "Can't you see I'm busy?! GET IT YOURSELF!"

After 11 p.m., I think they become blank-eyed zombies. Sometimes they don't even acknowledge me.

The labor and delivery ward — or "The House of Scream" as we sometimes call it — is another story. Upon entering this ward, I'm usually greeted by the cries of women in the midst of painful labor. Of course, I don't mind inserting epidurals in mothers-to-be during the day. But what bothers me is when a woman refuses an epidural early on because she's made a commitment to natural childbirth and then she finds the pain unendurable at the wretched hour of 3 a.m. By this point, the patient's cervix is well dilated and she's experiencing severe contractions occurring every two minutes.

What would have been a simple procedure becomes far more difficult and dangerous as I must try and insert a large, sharp and potentially paralyzing epidural needle into the back of the laboring woman, centimeters from the spinal cord, in between the contractions and screams of pain — and to do so on a moving target. Though I empathize with the woman attempting natural childbirth, at this late hour, with the risks involved, you can understand why I become a little miffed with her earlier decision to wait.

The vast majority of birthing experiences are happy and uncomplicated, resulting in a perfect baby for the overjoyed parents. However, there are some situations that aren't so positive for the future mom or dad.

It can be very difficult for the new dads-to-be. Their faces are sometimes filled with perspiration and panic as they sympathetically anticipate and experience each contraction with their partner. Unfortunately, the man can also become the focus of all the rage, frustration and pain that the woman experiences: "YOU did this to me. . . . How can YOU understand what I'm going through! . . ." I've heard unmentionable curses and abuses hurled at the poor guy, who only wants to be there and be supportive to his partner.

I've changed my routine and no longer allow the man to stay and hold the hand of his partner while I insert the epidural. In my mind's eye, I can still see the man's ashen face, his eyes rolling up into his head. He moans that he doesn't feel too well just before he faints with a dull thud beside the bed. The nurses and I have to try and catch him early, before he loses consciousness and becomes a patient himself.

"Honey, honey, are you okay?" the woman asks, trying to get a glimpse of her partner, as his head starts to sink towards the floor.

"He's going to be okay. Just needs a little fresh air," says the labor room nurse, as she helps the disorientated man to his feet.

"He's okay, isn't he?" she again asks.

"He'll be fine! I'm just going to help him out of the room. Now you just concentrate on being still with the doctor!" says the nurse as she assists the man out of the room.

"Now just be still. Don't move! I'm about to put the needle in," I remind her, again for the fifth time.

"ow, ow! I can feel another contraction coming! I CAN'T be still!" She screams for the sixth time, as she sways to and fro.

Sigh. Here we go again, I think to myself.

After having met so many people as they face sudden illness, it's tempting to automatically classify them and believe I can predict their behavior. But being on call teaches you to abandon your biases and judge each person as an individual.

One night, the surgeon called to say that a patient — let's call him Mr. B. — needed an operation to remove a bullet from his thigh after a drug deal gone bad. Mr. B. was stable and was being prepared for surgery.

"By the way, he's got no health insurance," the surgeon added, in a tired and frustrated tone, indicating that we would be providing charity medical service this late night. If I ever hoped to be paid, I would have go to Mr. B. directly. In a big city hospital, you resign yourself to the reality that even when it's late at night and you're fatigued and hungry, you will not always be paid for your services.

Many doctors gripe about universal health care, but from

a billing standpoint I think it's great. Stories about the old days abound, like having to personally bill each patient with no guarantee of getting paid or even having to barter for payment — "How about two chickens for an anesthetic?" Today, doctors just send the necessary information about the patient and surgery to the government or insurance group with the expectation that payment will follow.

Each year, more and more people enter the city, working under the radar, seeking anonymity. For various reasons, they shun and reject the support systems offered — like health insurance.

If the person is destitute or clearly just eking out a living, you just accept the situation and do your job. But, very occasionally, you sense that a patient may have the means to pay for health services and so you inquire about compensation. What risk is there in asking?

With low expectations, I went down to the emergency room to visit Mr. B.

As I approached a room in the distant area of the emergency department, I was immediately stopped at the doorway by two very large human towers dressed in black — one who resembled Andre the Giant and the other who looked like the brother of Shaquille O'Neal.

"What do you want?" the giant growled.

"I'm looking for Mr. B.," I squeaked, regretting more and more my decision to come.

From within the room, a raspy voice called out, "Let him in."

As I entered, I couldn't help but notice two very sleek,

scantily dressed and stunningly beautiful women, sitting cross-legged in mini-skirts on either side of the bed — my eyes followed their shapely thighs towards the mesmerizing curves of their torsos. And sitting between them, with a large bandage wrapped around his right thigh, was a small man in dark glasses. Reams of gold jewelry glistened around his neck and multiple rings shined on his fingers. I drew a deep breath, gathered courage and said, "Mr. B., I understand that you don't have any insurance, and I've just come here to tell you that there is a charge for anesthetic services."

He regarded me silently for some time and then took his glasses off. His face was not at all what I expected. He looked like a thoughtful man, and his brown eyes expressed a quiet intelligence. His breathing was slow and measured, and he pursed his lips as he studied me.

And he knew me. He understood my uneasiness as I approached a drug dealer for whom the normal rules didn't apply — a man who didn't have to pay, who could blow me off at any time and, with a gesture, have his guards eject me from his room.

He suddenly straightened up, sat erect and decreed, "Don't worry; Mr. B. is good for it. I'm a man of my word." And as he said this, his face was a mixture of defiance and honor, while he pointed a thumb in a clenched fist at his chest.

I thanked him and, with much relief, rushed out of the room.

The surgery proceeded smoothly.

To be frank, I really didn't believe that Mr. B. would pay me. There are no practical options to seek compensation in these situations. Credit agencies have no sway. Letters from lawyers emphasizing the serious legal consequences that would follow non-payment are of course, laughable.

However, the next day, I gathered my courage, and decided to make my way to Mr. B.'s room after surgery. Again standing on either side of the entrance were the large bodyguards. I asked for admission, and his voice ushered me in. The two breathtakingly exotic and beautiful women were closely nestled beside him as he recovered in bed. I asked him how he felt — everything was fine and, according to him, I had done a good job.

There was silence. He then looked me straight in the eyes and asked, "How much?"

I quoted him the fee: $200. He slowly reached into the pocket of his embroidered robe and pulled out a very large roll of hundred-dollar bills. He slowly counted and then handed me the money.

I thanked him again, and, as I started to leave, he spoke, his voice full of dignity and pride — "I told you not to worry. Mr. B. is a man of his word."

Staying Human

I have to admit I sometimes become jaded about illness and even death. This is not uncommon amongst people who are involved in high-stress, life-and-death situations. It's a defense mechanism that allows you to distance yourself from the sadness. Getting personally involved with every patient is exhausting. Like firemen, policemen and other healthcare workers, we depersonalize the situation. Conversations are filled with grim humor. The whole situation becomes coldly clinical.

However, events occur sometimes that re-humanize us, creating a strong connection to certain patients. These episodes happen, oftentimes not during the operation itself, but just before and after. The following cases illustrate some of these occasions.

It's 4 p.m. and the orthopedic surgeon has been asked to fix the broken hip of Mrs. Krakow. He tells me that even though she's only 50 years old, she has breast cancer that has spread throughout her body. The cancer has invaded her liver, causing metabolic poisons and bile to accumulate in her blood so that her skin and even the whites of her eyes are stained with a yellow hue. The metabolic toxins have caused her to become confused. The cancer has spread to her bones, making them so brittle that a simple fall can cause her hip to break like a toothpick.

He tells me this to reassure me that Mrs. Krakow's hip will not be fixed tonight or any night in the future. He considers her too high a risk for surgery: her body cannot metabolize drugs; her risk of significant blood loss during surgery is too great. She will die soon.

As he walks away, my pager rings. It's Mrs. Krakow's family doctor. He apologizes for paging me but explains that despite her condition, he still would like me to see her and assess if there is even a small possibility that her hip can be repaired. I reluctantly agree to see her, though I am secretly in agreement with the assessment of the orthopedic surgeon.

On the ward, a review of Mrs. Krakow's medical records verifies the bleak picture. Her room is located at the end of the old section of the hospital. As I wearily trudge down the long, time-worn corridor to her room, I hear my steps resonate off its bleached walls.

Her room is dark, small and stuffy. A very small window faces onto the brick wall of the adjacent building. To my left, I see her. I'm surprised she is not lying in bed but is sitting up despite what must be terrible pain in her broken hip. She is struggling to gaze out the window from her bed. As she turns her head, I see that her face is large and puffy, the result of steroids used to slow the cancer. Her hair is thin and wispy and there are bald spots scattered throughout her scalp — the signs of punishing failed chemotherapy regimes. She has large, yellow-stained eyes that almost bulge out of her face. In the corners of her eyes I can see the reflection of the dim overhead lights. I realize her eyes are filled with tears.

I explain to her that I've come to assess her candidacy for surgery. As the tears glisten in her eyes, she immediately interrupts me and speaks forcefully, her voice a mix of determination and urgency. I quickly realize that she is not confused at all. She is fully aware of her situation.

I'm caught off guard as she pleads to have the surgery. She knows that she has terminal cancer, that the cancer has spread throughout her body and that she only has a short time to live. She has no immediate family. She has vowed to get out of the hospital and be as independent as she possibly can be.

Before her accident, she was outside every day despite her weakness and fatigue. She would go shopping every day. It was during one of these outings to the supermarket that she fell and broke her hip. Now, she is a prisoner in this room. Her only view of the outside world has been the bricks of the adjacent building from the small window in her room.

For the last two days, she had been evaluated by numerous specialists and she realizes that she has only a small chance of receiving an assessment favorable to surgery. I can see the desperation in her eyes as she pleads with me for the surgery despite the high risks involved. She tells me she does not want to die in this bed. She wants to be able to walk outside again and feel the sun.

I try to assure her that I will attempt to convince the surgeon to perform the operation. I am aware that she is a high-risk patient, and that she may not survive the surgery or the recovery period afterwards.

As I make my way from the ward, I feel so ashamed. I had come to assess Mrs. Krakow like a medical bureaucrat, to certify the hopelessness of her situation and deny surgery — in effect, to sign her death certificate. She had ripped the cold clinical mask from my face. She had nothing to hide — no hidden agendas, no deception — she was simply requesting one last chance for happiness before death.

The image of this poor lady facing death while trapped in a miserable room, desperate to get out — her face and eyes, her thoughts and voice echoing in my head — had affected me deeply. I knew she had to be helped.

Catch-22

It's 1 a.m. and Dr. James Smith is calling me. He is a large, burly man, in his early 60s. His face has begun to show the effects of a long surgical career — furrowed brow and permanent creases between his eyes, a reflection of his cynicism after years of practice. He is a stubborn man with a contrarian streak. He would definitely go left if you told him to go right. His gruff demeanor is in no way a reflection of his surgical skill — his large hands move with the delicacy and grace of a skilled painter, every movement a marvel of precision and purpose. He's had years of experience as a surgeon and has probably seen every operative scenario imaginable.

Everyone knows that Dr. Smith will be retiring soon. His practice is slowly winding down and he is counting the last of his on-call days, like a prisoner anticipating the remaining days of incarceration. His operating philosophy is simple — avoid surgery if at all possible, especially if it has the potential to get you into trouble.

"Hi Paul. I just want to get your opinion about this guy that the intensive care doc is trying to get me to operate on … and I don't want to operate on him! The patient's name is Fallis, and he was operated on two weeks ago for a perforated intestine [literally, a hole in the gut]. He's got a terrible history — diabetes, drug addiction, heavy smoker with lung disease and recurrent pancreatitis. He was doing fine and was let out on a day pass today, and now he's suddenly had to come back in the hospital. He's in the intensive care being ventilated and they're having trouble keeping his oxygen levels up and his blood pressure — it's only about 70 and he's on big-time drugs just to keep it there. His blood sugars are way out of whack and his kidneys aren't working. He's a very high risk for surgery, don't you think?"

I try to focus and shake the fatigue out of my eyes. It has already been a very long day, with numerous cases that seemed to go nonstop throughout the night.

"Yeah, I think he'd definitely be a high-risk patient who might die on the table," I say.

"That's what I wanted to hear! Okay, thanks. I'll tell the intensive care doc that there's no way I'm doing this case. Bye."

I sit down thinking. "Fallis, Fallis? I remember that name!" Suddenly it all came back to me. Two weeks ago I had worked with another surgeon who cut out the leaking hole in Mr. Fallis's intestine and reattached the cut ends together. I remembered how Mr. Fallis had entered the operating room that day. Only 49 years old, the corrosive effects of years of drug abuse, poor nutrition and life as a street person had taken its toll and punished his body. He was rail thin, and had the look of a starving man 20 years older — hollowed cheeks, ghost-like complexion and thinning white hair. The ribs on his chest resembled those of a cadaver and the fingers of his right hand were stained with nicotine. I recalled the look of pain and fear in his eyes as we transferred him to the operating table. We tried to reassure him that everything would work out fine. The surgery proceeded uneventfully and it seemed to us that with his gut fixed, he could perhaps eventually heal. But given his poor physical status, the recovery would be very long and difficult.

What I recall most is the notation on the computer as I reviewed his medical history prior to surgery: "Has a 13-year-old son."

It isn't standard practice to include personal information like that in a list of medical problems. It changed my viewpoint of Mr. Fallis — not just a lifelong drug abuser and street person, but in fact, a man with a family. It also brought things into personal perspective — I have a 13-year-old son.

I want to know how he had become so quickly and critically ill again. And so I call the intensive care doctor working that night. I am happy to hear that Dr. Fine is working tonight. His compact figure, kind face and understated and quiet manner veil an imposing clinical acumen and wry sense of humor. As I've discussed previously, as far as clinical skills are concerned, there are "good" and "bad" doctors. David is definitely in the "good" camp. Because he is an excellent diagnostician and clinician, I know that any patient would have the best possible care under Dr. Fine.

He is also a reasonable person. He knows when to treat patients with high-powered drugs and techniques to try and save them, and when to gently discuss with their relatives the fact that taking heroic measures would only prolong the patient's suffering. He knows when it would be merciful to let that person go peacefully.

"David, what's going on with Mr. Fallis?" I ask.

"Well, he was out today for the first time since his initial operation. It's his wife's birthday. He was walking when he suddenly had abdominal pain and collapsed. He's got a 13-year-old son, you know."

"I know," I reply, reminded again of my own son. "I was involved with his initial surgery."

Dr. Fine pauses. "I put a tube down his airway and have got him on the ventilator. I've got Levophed infusing into him to maintain his blood pressure. He's very sick but I've got him stabilized as best I can. I really think his anastomosis [the previous intestinal repair] has fallen apart."

If this is the case, it means that feces are now leaking directly into Mr. Fallis's abdomen. The highly toxic bacteria from the bowel will create a septic infection in the bloodstream with toxins affecting all organs of the body. The lungs will fail to oxygenate the blood, the kidneys will start to shut down and the heart will fail.

"If that's the case," I say, "then his only hope is to get that anastomosis fixed. Is that what you think, David?"

"Yes," replies Dr. Fine. "James is refusing to operate, saying that Fallis is too sick to withstand the operation. . . . James doesn't want to kill him in order to try and fix problems that I can't 100 percent prove are there. James says Fallis could be septic from another source, like pneumonia, and he could have recurrent pancreatitis as well."

I am immediately filled with guilt. When James called me earlier he only gave me the basic sketch of Mr. Fallis's grave condition, not mentioning the possible postsurgical breakdown of the anastomosis. I had agreed with him that there was a high possibility of intra-operative death, given the clinical story he'd given me. But I now feel I had been misled to concur with James' desire to not get involved.

On the other hand, I understand the enormous responsibility and pressure he must have felt as the surgeon on call. This decision is the ultimate life-or-death Catch-22. Should the surgeon operate in order to save a life, knowing that the stress of the operation may kill the patient? Or should the surgeon wait until the patient is "optimized" and stabilized, knowing that optimization may never occur? In this case, the patient could die before the operation.

"Should I call another surgeon to operate?" I can hear the hint of desperation and exasperation in his voice.

"No, you just can't do that, David. You know that James is on call and is the responsible physician. Anyways, the other surgeons would repeat what I just said in the first place and refuse to come in. And you know James — if you were to try to push him, he'd just stick his heels in the ground, and you would get nowhere!"

There is a long pause and then a sigh from Dr. Fine. "Well, I'll just have to stabilize him the best I can and hope that he hangs on until the next surgeon begins his call. Thanks for calling, Paul."

I look at my watch. It is 1:30 in the morning. The next surgeon will begin his or her day of call at around seven in the morning, after receiving a report from James about patients seen during his shift.

Later in the morning, at 7:15, I go to the cafeteria. I definitely need a strong cup of coffee to stay awake. Throughout the early morning, the labor and delivery ward had kept me busy with requests for epidurals. Any thoughts of Mr. Fallis have long since been pushed back during the busy hours of the morning. But as I pour coffee, Dr. Fine walks into the cafeteria. For a brief moment we glance at each other and then look away. Seeing Dr. Fine immediately brings to mind the frustration and helplessness of our earlier conversation. We then both walk towards the cashier with our coffees.

"How is Mr. Fallis doing?" I ask.

His weary face meets mine. He hesitates, and then in a soft voice replies, "He died around 4:30 this morning."

"Oh," I reply, as my faint hope is replaced with guilt-tinged anger and disappointment.

"Too bad he just couldn't hang on a bit longer. The operation might have saved him."

"Yes, it might have," I say.

There is a pause, and then we part. And all the while, as I trudge up the stairs to the locker room, wearily pull off my O.R. greens and even as I leave the hospital, I can only think about Mr. Fallis and his 13-year-old son.

CHAPTER 3

Off-Label Truths About Doctors

Examining the Specialists

There are so many specialties in medicine today. Medical practice has become broad and diverse. Each specialist has only a general idea about what really happens in other areas of specialization. An orthopedic surgeon knows little about the challenges facing a plastic surgeon and vice versa. The only opportunity most doctors have to learn about other specialties is during brief one- or two-week stints while at medical school — and that's not sufficient to really understand what goes on.

Even after graduation, most doctors work in a kind of isolation from their colleagues, unaware of how others practice. They're too busy to observe other doctors at work, and even if they had the opportunity to do so, many fear they will lose face and appear insecure in their abilities.

In the operating room, I get to work with all the surgeons.

Ironically, instead of directly asking another surgeon, they will ask me — "Paul, just how does Dr. So-and-So do this operation? Does he use this or that instrument? Does he use this particular technique?" When new techniques are introduced, even at large national and international meetings and medical conferences, it is up to each doctor to adopt or reject the new techniques; these decisions are left to the individual.

As an anesthetist, I also consult with internists (doctors specializing in internal medicine) and other non-surgical colleagues as we evaluate patients for upcoming operations. I also work with gastroenterologists, radiologists and cardiologists to provide sedation for treatments and tests.

With this unique, broad exposure other specialists don't have, anesthetists understand — and tolerate — the quirks and personalities of many specialists.

Do doctors within a specialty have a common personality profile? Are the personalities of orthopedic surgeons different from those of cardiologists? The answer to both questions is yes.

In order to understand this, let's see if the personality of medical students influences the specialties they'll choose. Are medical students drawn to a specialty because the specific requirements match their personalities? In his book *The Ultimate Guide to Choosing a Medical Specialty*, Dr. Brian Freeman summarizes research confirming the relationship between personality and choice of specialty. P. Zeidow, in his paper published in *Academic Medicine*, argued that aggressive, confident and competitive students who seek immediate solutions were drawn to the surgical specialties. Introverts, and especially those who had undergone psychotherapy, were most likely to become psychiatrists. Students who felt more secure in structured environments characterized by technical routines were drawn towards the hospital specialties, like anesthesiology and radiology.

In another paper, Ronald J. Makert analyzed the results of a psychological test called "The Big Five" to measure the five dimensions of personality — neuroticism, extroversion, openness, agreeableness and conscientiousness — in medical students. His research revealed that the least agreeable and most judgmental students leaned towards surgical specialties. Those who were the most open to new ideas and possessed a non-judgmental manner opted for psychiatry. Finally, those exhibiting both neuroticism and a need to gather information became internists.

The relationship of personality and specialty makes perfect sense. For example, if you were on the operating table rapidly bleeding to death, you would want a surgeon who would seize control, coldly look at the facts without an excessive display of emotion, make a rapid, self-assured judgment and decisively solve the problem.

Now imagine a surgeon with the personality of a psychiatrist in this emergency setting. He or she would want to gradually assess the facts, looking for connections and meaning. Despite the urgency of the situation, he or she might be overly concerned about how decisions affect others in the room or how others feel about them, resulting in hesitation. This is not the kind of thinking you want if you're bleeding out.

If a psychiatrist who thought like a surgeon gave psychotherapy, he or she would impatiently listen with preconceived notions of normal behavior. The psychiatrist with the surgeon's personality traits would quickly and analytically diagnose a specific mental disorder and probably tell the patient that he or she is crazy. A prescription would be given to immediately correct the "imbalance." This approach is obviously inappropriate for a psychiatrist.

The Test

What are the personality characteristics within a specialty? In Dr. Freeman's book, he describes the Myers-Briggs Type Indicator — a psychological test based on Carl Jung's theory of personality — that helps describe personality in four basic dimensions. Research has revealed some combinations of these four factors in each specialty. Using these results, I'll show the common Myers-Briggs indicators found in each specialty.

The first factor defines how you relate to others — as *extrovert (E)* versus *introvert (I)*.

The second concerns how you take in information. Do you only value and use information taken in by your *senses (S),* or do you use your senses to look for connections and relationships, i.e., are you an *intuitive (N)* thinker?

The third concerns how decisions are made. Do you draw conclusions objectively, based on logical *thinking (T),* or do you rely on subjective thoughts, empathy and *feelings (F)?*

Finally, what kind of life do you want to lead? Is it orderly, scheduled and predictable so that you are *judgmental (J)?* Or are you more open-minded, allowing other views to percolate in your mind as you think the world should be openly *perceived (P)?*

Got it? Let's go.

Orthopedic Surgeons

Most orthopedic surgeons are extroverts (E) who objectively act on what their senses (S) tell them; they are rational thinkers (T), with some leading lives that can be rigidly judgmental (J), while others, outside of work, want to perceive (P) and experience as much as possible.

There is a well-known joke orthopedic surgeons like to tell: a long line of people are patiently waiting to enter the pearly gates of heaven. Suddenly, someone in a white lab coat pushes his way forward from the back of the line. He forces the gates open and strides through. One of the people in line turns and asks the person behind, "Who was that?" The person replies, "That was God. Some days He likes to pretend He's an orthopedic surgeon."

This male-dominated specialty attracts those whose attitude is "If something is broken, we can fix it." This is a "macho" specialty. If you predicted which toddlers were most likely to become orthopedic surgeons, you'd be safe betting on the boys with toy tools who push other children out of their path. They would be focused on pulling apart and rebuilding the playground.

During my medical training, I recall the orthopedic staff person and his residents swaggering through the hallways of the hospital. Their voices would bellow politically incorrect jokes or last night's football and hockey scores. I would not hear them discussing last night's performance of *Swan Lake*. Some residents imitated this masculine persona so as not to jeopardize completion of the program.

This high-testosterone personality must pervade into the

bedroom. In a physician survey, orthopedic surgeons admitted to — or perhaps bragged about — having the most frequent sex per week.

Their cars are typically expensive, high-powered performance machines. They'll rarely be seen driving a gas-sipping Prius or a humble van.

There's no fiddling with pills, injections or psychotherapy during their work. The tools of the orthopedic surgeon are the hammer, screwdriver, drill, cement and wire — mixed with a lot of testosterone-fuelled muscle and sweat. Watching a major orthopedic operation is like observing a construction project, complete with the sounds of drilling, hammering and sawing and the smell of chemical cements. In fact, the drills, hammers and power saws orthopedic surgeons use are remarkably similar to those used by a contractor. In many ways, it's like watching an episode of *Holmes on Homes*.

Most work the orthopedic surgeon does is the antithesis of delicate and tiny. A limb is not carefully moved into position; it's grabbed, pulled, braced and secured for the cut of the scalpel. Their operating tools are larger than those of other specialties — oversized sharp blades, big pincers and huge graspers. They are designed to open, expose and hold large bones as quickly and firmly as possible. The bone is scraped, chiseled and pinned into position.

These types of operations inflict a great deal of wear and tear on the instruments. When surgeons from other specialties find their instruments broken and bent, they'll half-jokingly ask, "Have the bone surgeons been using my instruments? Don't let them use my stuff again."

For bigger operations, like a knee replacement, a large number of specialized tools and components are needed. All together, they remind me of a huge, intricate Mechano Set.

While vigorously hammering components into the leg, it's not uncommon for the surgeon to be completely unaware of the fact he has sprayed blood onto the O.R. lights and even onto the ceiling. In no way does this mean the work is done without care. Each cut, drill and shaving must be precise, because misalignments can be a disaster — possibly resulting in a patient who can't walk normally.

An orthopedic surgeon's sensitivity to the "feminine side" is very low. Though I know some women who have become orthopedic surgeons, they are few and far between. Many of them have had very difficult times in this male-dominated training program. Some were under tremendous pressure to quit, because it was thought they were not tough enough for the program. They persevered with a lot of guts and determination.

As far as life outside of the operating room is concerned, orthopedic surgeons are split into two groups, confirmed by the Myers-Briggs results. Some orthopedic surgeons maintain a very rigid, scheduled life outside of the operating room. Others have a more relaxed and spontaneous existence, as they open their lives to as much personal experience as possible.

General Surgeons

Most general surgeons are extroverts (E), though they are less extroverted than orthopedic surgeons; they accept only objective clinical sensory input (S), make decisions based on objective, rational thinking (T) and are more close-minded, scheduled and judgmental (J) in life.

There are many problems a general surgeon must face every day. For them, being the decision maker — the boss in control — is important. It's about using your own hands to make an immediate positive difference in someone's life.

For general surgeons, their principal area of practice involves the organs of the abdomen, the abdominal wall and the breast. Most frequently, a general surgeon operates upon the gallbladder, stomach, appendix, intestines, hernias and the breasts. Many things can go wrong with these parts of the body — from cancers and blockages to swellings and infections.

General surgeons revel in their mastery and understanding of all organs found in the body cavity. They feel in their element when using their skills to explore and repair damaged organs.

These days, more surgery is being converted from open operations into keyhole surgery. Small incisions, less than half an inch wide, are made through the abdominal wall and mini-cameras and pincer-like instruments are inserted. The surgeon operates while watching a video screen of the operating area. It's like playing a video game. In fact a recent study has shown that video gamers have an advantage in mastering these key-hole surgeries as compared to non-gamers. Another study has shown up to four percent of trainees will never master keyhole techniques. Some don't have the ability to safely manipulate instruments in the body while watching a video display.

General surgeons must occasionally work in extremely gross and disgusting situations, when blockages occur in the intestines. Growths, swellings or twists cause gases and feces to accumulate and expand within the intestines. The intestines can resemble a giant snake; I've seen a case where the intestines were almost as thick as a man's thigh and a meter in length.

I'll admit it's impressive to see the glistening, almost velvety yards of pink-grey intestines that almost spill out of the wound. Like a silky, giant worm, the intestines contract on their own and squirm as they are manipulated, cut and sewn by the experienced hands of the surgeon.

The scene reminds me of an episode from *Alien* as I look down at the sleeping patient's face and see the gas-filled tube arising from the open abdomen — the accumulation of fecal material, half-digested food and gases that have sometimes been trapped for days. When the surgeon cuts the intestines open and releases the gases, the terrible smells in the operating room can be suffocating. People rush to spray deodorizing aerosols into the air or onto their masks to cover the odors. The doors in the O.R. are temporarily flung open for better ventilation. Any thoughts of grabbing a quick snack after the operation are quickly squelched. A general surgeon may work under conditions like these, starting late into the night or into the early hours of the morning.

Other surgeries are upsetting for different reasons. When an operation on a young person unexpectedly reveals that cancer has spread, it is a death sentence, and the mood in the operating room changes. What started out as a typical day — filled with banter and humor — becomes quiet and somber. The surgeon explores the abdominal cavity, feeling for the hard cancer nodules on the liver, lymph nodes and other organs — assessing the potential complications the cancer will create.

There is a mistaken impression that modern diagnostic

screening before surgery — ultrasound, CAT scans, MRIs — can reveal tumor spread before the operation. This is not always true. Studies have shown that metastases — the spread of tumor cells — can go undetected, so the real extent of cancer spread is only revealed during an operation. In surgery as in life, no matter how much you test and plan, the outcome is not always predictable.

The surgery becomes *palliative*: not done to cure but as a way to improve the quality of remaining life, or to help extend life a little. It allows a person to eat, drink or breathe normally for as long as possible, before the cancer kills.

Most general surgeons are overworked, enduring gruelling hours for lower pay than other specialists. They whine about this fact over and over again. However, if you ask them if they love their job, most say they do. In truth, though the work is hard, they love cutting, suturing and solving surgical problems.

Urologists

The majority of urologists are Introverts (I) who rely on clinical objective sensations at work (S) while basing decisions on subjective feelings (F); in life, they are perceivers (P) who want to experience as much as possible.

In general, urologists are a professionally content and happy group. They are the surgical group with the lowest divorce rate. They receive regular ribbing about working with urine, the penis and prescribing Viagra, and they tend to accept this with tolerance and humor.

Most enjoy their work and interact very well with their

patients. There are two reasons for this. First, most urologists are men and because they are dealing with sexual function and urination — very personal subjects for most men — they become not just doctors but confidantes. They show a great deal of sensitivity and understanding when remedying these problems. Most urologists talk to their patients in a friendly and personal manner, addressing them by their first names. I've noticed the contrast with specialists in other fields, who address their patients formally, using only surnames. Second, most of their patients don't have life-threatening diseases, and the treatments available to solve urination and sexual problems are quite effective. Their patients are very grateful. This gives urologists a great deal of job satisfaction.

Outside of the hospital, urologists have varied interests, are open-minded and like to travel.

There are interesting procedures urologists perform on what I call "penis day," and as the name suggests, these involve the male organ of worship and envy. These can be a series of circumcisions performed on both children and adults, in which the foreskin is removed because it has contracted and squeezed the tip of the penis, making urination difficult. Other operations involve the correction of severe left or right deviations of the penis that occur during an erection. It's caused by the development of scar tissue and named Peyronie's Disease — or what I call the "Clinton" sign because of a trait supposedly revealed during the Monica Lewinsky scandal. With the patient under anesthetic, the urologist first wraps a tight rubber band around the base of the penis. He inflates the penis by injecting saline into large penile veins, causing an erection. Close and careful observation of the resultant bend occurs. Fibrous scars in the connective tissue that envelops the penis is removed. Things straighten out.

In another operation, the penile vein is ligated (tied) to prevent blood from leaving the penis, helping men with penile dysfunction maintain an erection. The test for success is done by again inflating the penis with saline to see if it remains at attention.

The penis, as it is alternately inflated to stand at attention and then released to become flaccid, resembles an inflatable dildo. In other words, at its basic mechanical level, a man's expression of sexual arousal and passion can be reduced to a simple hydraulic action.

As I've said before, many men coming into the O.R. have such good relationships with their urologists that they are comfortable discussing their penile problems in front of other staff. I recall one elderly gentleman who needed a circumcision. Immediately upon entering the O.R., he lifted up his gown, exposing his penis to the entire room. Vigorously simulating lovemaking with his penis and hand, he boldly said to the urologist, "Doc, this is the piece of skin that rubs when I make love to my wife, and it catches, you know, pulls and hurts here." A rookie scrub nurse stood speechless, her eyes fixed on the gentleman's display. To me, it was as if he had leisurely entered a barbershop with the instructions, "Tony, take a little off the sides, but leave the top long."

Psychiatrists
Most psychiatrists are introverts (I); they organize information

looking for connections, relationships and intuition (N), and they base conclusions upon sensitivity and feelings (F).

A psychiatrist at a teaching center confirmed that 10 to 15 percent of psychiatric residents entered the program because they believe themselves to be a little crazy, and want to confirm this suspicion. As mentioned before, many medical students entering this specialty have undergone psychotherapy.

Psychiatrists are very interesting people. You notice, outwardly at least, they seem happy. (However, you also wonder if this is just a sham to hide some very dark unresolved issues ... just kidding.) Most psychiatrists can converse on a number of subjects — from wine and music to literature and travel. They have eclectic tastes and are the best people to invite to parties. They have the ability to keep conversations rolling with such phrases as, "Well, what do *you* think about that?"

They are very thoughtful people and perhaps over-analyze faults in their own lives a little too deeply. A study published in the *New England Journal of Medicine* showed psychiatrists have the highest divorce rate of the specialties, approaching 50 percent.

According to a paper by I. Berman published in *Academic Medicine*, 50 percent of psychiatrists believe other medical specialists view their work as less important. They are right: many other specialists believe the treatment of mental illness is ineffective, despite the fact that studies have shown psychiatrists are very successful in treating many mental disorders. Psychiatrists are the Rodney Dangerfields of the specialists' world.

Plastic Surgeons

No other specialty illustrates how medicine can be an art as well as a science. A good plastic surgeon not only has to be technically good, but must also achieve a standard of beauty that is pleasing to the eyes of both patient and surgeon.

Most plastic surgeons have egos that are a bit inflated. It's understandable given that many of them interact with the rich, famous and beautiful people. They must market and sell themselves in order to attain a certain profile in a profession that's becoming more competitive and crowded.

The patients of plastic surgeons often experience "transference" — the process by which emotions and desires originally associated with one person are unconsciously shifted to the surgeon. Some have told me there are always opportunities to accept this transference, especially after the surgery is successful, and the grateful patient wishes to have a relationship that's beyond doctor and patient. One plastic surgeon told me how he evaluated the consequences of giving in to such temptations. "I always think about the terrible things this would do to my family, my practice and the patient if I were to get involved. I've seen what happens to others. Why would I do that to my life?"

Many plastic surgeons have a unique patient profile. For example, a surgeon may start practice with a few strippers or dancers who want breast enlargements. If he does a good job, word spreads in that community. More of these women come for breast enlargement and eventually much of his practice is this type of surgery. The same is true about rhinoplasty, where word has spread that Dr. X is the best for nose jobs.

On the other hand, many plastic surgeons admit they don't want to be known to have only one type of client. One surgeon confessed she rejected a man who had just finished his sex-change hormone therapy and wanted cosmetic surgery. She told him she was not qualified to do this kind of surgery when, in fact, her reservations were based on her desire not to have a practice full of only one kind of patient.

The type of surgery performed changes with the age of the patient. A surgeon whose practice focuses predominantly on abdominoplasty (tightening of the stomach wall), liposuction and breast-enlargement told me most of his patients are a certain age. At this time in their lives, breasts and abdomens are the major concern. "But as my patients grow older and their faces wrinkle, I'll be doing their facelifts. Then this will be my most frequent operation."

An excellent plastic surgeon is meticulous from start to finish — precisely marking lines on the skin to cut, folding and stretching the skin as he or she works, like an artisan creating a masterpiece. Skin is remarkably elastic and can be stretched to an incredible degree when separated from underlying tissues. The excess skin is cut off and the edges carefully and precisely sutured, so wrinkles and folds magically disappear.

Certain things the plastic surgeon does remind me of an artist who invites others to assess his work. When he is almost finished with a breast augmentation, he will ask me to sit the sleeping patient up until almost completely upright. There, in the cloistered privacy of the operating room, the O.R. team is invited to stand at the foot of the bed to comment and suggest improvements: ". . . very natural looking, but don't you think the right breast should be little bit higher? What do you think about the size? Do the nipples look natural? Do you think 350cc of saline per breast is out of proportion to her body?" After we have made our suggestions and the surgeon is satisfied that he has done his best, I flatten the bed again. He meticulously sutures, ensuring that no suture lines will appear when the patient has healed.

Anesthetists

Most anesthetists are introverts (I) who only accept objective clinical sensory (S) information and base decisions on personal, subjective feelings (F).

Most anesthetists are very comfortable being "behind the scenes" people and are not looking to be the center of attention. Anesthetists are satisfied to let others in the operating room bask in the limelight and accept the praise.

I'll admit most of us don't have outstanding communication skills. You might expect this from someone who says "I'm going to put you to sleep" a lot of the time. In reality, anesthetists communicate well to patients on a clinical rather than an emotional level. It's easy to review medical histories before operations. Detailed interviews occur during consultations, when possible operative complications are investigated.

The real deficit is in emotional intelligence, where there is a problem of self- and social-awareness. This might be related to the frequent introversion seen in psychological tests. Even outside the hospital, we typically pursue individual or small-group activities. We're a pretty boring group — definitely not the life of the party.

We're also pretty lousy dressers. When large groups of

anesthetists gather at national conventions, you'll notice people wearing the dreariest, most mismatched and unfashionable clothes. It's because our work clothes are the O.R. greens. We anesthetists don't have to dress in a suit, tie or fancy dress, because our office is the operating room. Other staff and patients don't care how we dress when we're not in our greens. Anesthetists' lack of a fashion sense relates to our introverted nature. *Haute couture* is definitely not a concern.

An article about specialists and pop culture showed that anesthetists spend more leisure time, compared to other specialists, looking at the internet and reading about world events and the stock market. More than other specialties, we also like to watch videos and movies.

While the vast majority of anesthetists like to stay in the background and just do a good job, there are a small number who are exceptions; they desire to be in the limelight and garner attention. That's difficult to do in the operating room. Because these people have good management skills, they assume administrative or leadership positions and try to get noticed. Some crave admiration and respect. Others promote themselves as experts or visionaries in the field. One anesthetist fancies himself the epitome of class and fairness, but his selfish and biased decisions betray him. We cringe when another egotistical fellow portrays himself as a refined upper-class sophisticate who uses every opportunity to end discussions with an insincere and pretentious "cheers."

There is a dark side to the specialty. Anesthetists are three times more likely than other doctors to abuse drugs. One reason is ease of access to powerful narcotics and tranquilizers, which are used daily during clinical practice. They have an intimate understanding of the pharmacology of each drug through their training and clinical experience. They feel they can regulate and control the side effects of each drug. Finally, introversion is a factor; they like the ability to self-administer and control their own sensory stimulation without the need of outside, social interaction.

Studies have shown anesthetists are at three times the risk of drug-related death and twice the risk of drug-related suicide as compared to other specialties. Also, once addicted, the rates of successful re-entry into the specialty are very poor.

During an operation, the anesthetist not only makes sure you go to sleep and wake up, but he or she tries to protect you from the stresses and rigors of surgery. While the surgeon is busy cutting and suturing, the anesthetists will make sure that you don't become dehydrated. He or she will transfuse blood if you bleed excessively as well as make sure your heart and kidneys don't become damaged. Anesthetists monitor your temperature to make sure you're kept warm. Pain medicines, nerve blocks and anti-vomit medicine are given, so that you don't wake up from the operation shivering, throwing up or screaming in pain.

Many people think that when one is anesthetized, the body is asleep. Actually, when the surgeon cuts, the body is still awake, though the mind is unaware. The blood pressure and heart rate will race higher and muscles contract as the body literally squirms and writhes to scream "ouch!" Powerful drugs must be given to control this stress response and to keep the body from jerking and moving during operations.

Gastroenterologists

I would describe most gastroenterologists as "you get what you see" types. Most act in a straightforward, direct manner. Many can be very gruff and surprisingly blunt. You'll be given frank opinions upfront.

They diagnose and solve problems of the digestive system. They enjoy procedures using fiberoptic scopes, probing deep into the digestive system for diagnosis and treatment.

Gastroenterologists are aware their specialty doesn't have the glamour, say, of cardiology. However, they know the digestive process is an important concern to all of us as we think about eating with every hunger pang, stomach gurgle and cramp.

I find their indifference to the smell and exposure of digestive secretions a bit disconcerting. Many times, I've seen gastroenterologists adjust their glasses and answer cell phones with secretion-covered gloves during a procedure — without hesitation or second-thoughts. I guess constant exposure in this line of work desensitizes you to the normal discomfort most of us would feel.

A recent paper published by a group of gastroenterologists has shown that the blood antibodies to *H. Pylori* (bacterium responsible for many stomach ulcers) was found more frequently in gastroenterologists as compared to the general population. This would mean gastroenterologists had been exposed to this bacterium. When I asked a gastroenterologist about these blood levels, he casually replied, "It's because we get the gut bacteria on our hands and clothes while we work, and then we inadvertently eat it. It gets into our gut and we develop antibodies to it." I can tell you since learning this, I try to confirm that gastroenterologists have washed their hands before I shake them.

Gastroenterologists see many patients who complain endlessly about their eating and digestive problems. For gastroenterologists, it can become a never-ending stream of complaints concerning every food-sensitivity imaginable. Thus, an invitation to eat with a group of gastroenterologists is an opportunity to join them as they escape all the digestive griping. It means you're going to enjoy the digestive process in all its basic, uninhibited and natural glory. Expect lots of good food with people who understand all its richness, value and pleasures that it brings.

A gastroenterologist carries out procedures involving long, snake-like scopes introduced through the mouth or anus. These "scoping" studies investigate and diagnose the cause of any unusual symptoms of the gut — like nausea, difficulty swallowing, cramping and pain. Unusual signs of weight loss, bleeding, abnormal bowel movements and abnormal laboratory results can be investigated by looking into the digestive tract. Diagnostic biopsies (samples) can be obtained through the scopes, with the aid of miniature loops, graspers and suction devices. Pre-cancerous polyps are removed to prevent cancers from developing.

The scope images are viewed on high definition video screens. Large, python-like flexible scopes, many feet in length, are inserted through the anus to examine the long intestines.

The images on the video screen, as the scope rapidly makes its way through the anus and into the intestines, resembles a virtual reality simulation at Disney World. One patient who saw his gut video described it as an amusement ride — Journey Through the Haunted Tunnel.

As you watch the screen, there is the sensation of being on a roller-coaster ride, rapidly ascending and descending into a twisting, dim, subterranean tunnel. The walls of the tunnel are lined with shiny irregular crevices and folds that fly by as you twist and turn. Occasionally, the ride is interrupted to stop and pick up samples or snip off mushroom-shaped growths, illuminated in corners of the tunnel. This simulated movement is so realistic certain people experience vertigo and motion sickness while watching.

Cardiologists

More introverted (I) than extroverted (E), cardiologists evaluate clinical information intuitively (N), looking for connections and relationships; they come to logical, thoughtful (T) conclusions.

Cardiologists have been compared to fighter pilots navigating through high-risk situations. They carry out critical, calculated strategies with expert precision.

This is a specialty that allows them to perform many important procedures. They analyze heart function by looking at ultrasound and nuclear scans of the beating heart. They can insert small stents (tubes) into the heart vessels, to increase blood flow and avert a possible heart attack. They can also deliver electrical shocks to the heart or use small wires to burn diseased areas within the heart in order to restore normal heartbeats.

Cardiologists are courted by the pharmaceutical companies to prescribe numerous drugs such as antihypertensive medicines; cholesterol-lowering medicines; blood thinners; and heart rhythm, anti-angina and heart-failure medicines.

Because the heart is so central to overall health and survival, serious conditions that affect it are naturally dramatic. In many cases, this focuses much attention towards the doctor who looks after this all-important organ. Cardiology is a glamorous specialty.

Of course, all this attention can produce a very big ego. Cardiologists consider themselves to be the kings of the non-surgical specialties. More often than not, they are the doctors who drive big black Mercedes. If you see a fellow in the hospital who radiates a sense of importance, and wears a tailored silk suit, Ralph Lauren shirt, Gucci shoes, with a stethoscope around his neck, he's most likely a cardiologist.

Of all the internal medicine subspecialties, cardiology boasts some of the highest median compensation.

Neurologists

Mostly introverts (I), neurologists take in clinical information and look for connections and relationships in an intuitive (N) manner.

Neurologists are obsessive-compulsive people. They have to be in order to be good at their job. Diagnosis is based on highly specialized and complex algorithms — a step-by-step clinical history and physical examination that lead down a diagnostic path, to evaluate a patient's brain function. In essence, a diagnosis is made by using history and physical examination, and by putting together the pieces of an intricate neuroanatomy puzzle in order to solve a medical mystery.

This obsessive-compulsive behavior is seen in many aspects of the neurologist's life. A cruel colleague I know will slightly move objects on the desk of a neurologist — watching the growing anxiety on the neurologist's face, as he unsuccessfully suppresses the urge to reposition them.

Unfortunately, even with the advances of science, most progressive, debilitating neurological diseases are not currently curable. In most cases, the treatments a neurologist can prescribe only help to alleviate symptoms of the disease. Most neurologists accept their status as specialists in the diagnosis of incurable disease.

Obstetrician and Gynecologists

The majority of OBGs are introverts (I) whose clinical evaluation is based on objective sensory (S) facts and whose conclusions are based upon objective, logical thinking (T); they live life in a planned, controlled and judgmental (J) manner.

Some surveys have shown that most obstetricians and gynecologists, though introverts, are very concerned with maintaining good outside appearances and impressions as a way of protecting their sensitive and emotional psyches.

They get joy and satisfaction through helping to bring a healthy baby into the world. At the same time, they must get used to the vomit, urine, feces, blood and amniotic fluid that come with delivery and birth.

Paradoxically, many surgeons act in a very condescending way towards obstetricians and gynecologists and will frequently criticize their surgical skills. When a surgeon is asked by an obstetrician and gynecologist to help out, it is not unusual for the surgeon to suggest and "teach" his or her colleague about proper techniques. During medical school, it was not uncommon to hear staff surgeons make derogatory comments about the surgical skills of obstetricians and gynecologists — comments like "they are not real surgeons." This is probably because most surgeons feel their long work hours, exposure to emergency and trauma makes them better in the operating room. It probably has a lot to do with the surgeons' critical and opinionated personalities as well.

When obstetricians first start to practice, they have a great deal of enthusiasm and excitement for their work. Obviously, sharing the success of delivering a baby with the family is very rewarding. However, you can't fail to notice that this enthusiasm wanes over the years. It's sad to see the previously energetic and happy face of the obstetrician become fatigued and jaded as time passes.

Obviously, sleep deprivation is a very large factor. Obstetricians and gynecologists spend many nights working long hours and being present for early morning deliveries. This results in interrupted and poor-quality sleep. Over the years, it takes its toll.

Furthermore, the current climate of hyper litigation puts tremendous pressure on obstetricians. They have the highest malpractice insurance premiums and the highest incidence of lawsuits during their careers as compared to other specialties. The expectation is, of course, for the delivery of a "perfect baby." Yet, even when an obstetrician takes all the precautions in prenatal care, with screening ultrasounds and other tests, and is available and prepared for unexpected events at delivery, a baby can be born with serious complications. Having this constant legal threat is taxing on a career.

Unfortunately, this stress may take its toll on their libidos. According to a survey, obstetricians and gynecologists are the least satisfied among all the specialists with their sex lives.

I know there will be protest from some specialists, who will totally disagree with my characterizations. Of course, there will be exceptions to the studies and opinions presented. But the majority of my colleagues will honestly admit that each specialty attracts a certain type of person — an individual whose personality is very similar to their own. As I've indicated, many specialties demand that a practitioner exhibit specific strengths in order to be able to thrive and cope with the demands of their jobs.

CHAPTER 4

The Good, the Bad and the Ugly

Entering Tiger Country

Dr. Huynh enters the operating room. Atop his long, lanky frame is a youthful, smiling face that that belies his status as a new, recently graduated staff person. After exchanging greetings and a few jokes with us, he puts his sterile operating room gown and gloves on. In the background can be heard sounds of the music on the radio, the anesthesia machine ventilator and the beeping pulse of the sleeping patient. He calmly reviews important instructions with the O.R. nurse, such as patient positioning, video camera placement and instrument positioning and settings. The team is now ready to begin the minimally invasive keyhole surgery to remove Mr. Smith's bowel cancer.

Throughout the surgery, there are no surprises. Dr. Huynh is in control. His hand movements are fluid and graceful as he moves instruments through the body wall into the patient's abdominal cavity, revealing the silken, glistening rolls of grey-pink guts, the dark purple liver and other major organs. The danger areas — "tiger country," as we call it — are identified and noted: major vessels and delicate organs that must be cautiously avoided.

On the video screen, seemingly endless loops of floppy bowel are pulled, teased and manipulated by the long pincer-like instruments used by the surgeon. Tissue plains and bowel layers are gently peeled apart or cut by the electrocautery probe. The cancer-filled section is removed and the resulting free ends of good bowel are quickly sewn together. Bleeding is minimal.

The whole operation is completed with precision and skill. From start to finish, it is a thing of beauty.

Dr. Huynh's stellar reputation preceded his work at our hospital. As a resident, others noted how quickly and easily he mastered the intricate challenges of keyhole surgery.

Like star athletes in the sports world, some doctors in the surgical specialties easily grasp concepts and master techniques. They see the whole operative field, and are aware of all the important organs, like a sports star who knows the position of all the players on the field. A gifted doctor knows all the movements and effects of his instruments, just like an athlete understands actions and reactions in the flow of a game. Their eye-hand coordination is excellent. They have almost an *innate ability* to position and manipulate droopy sutures for tying knots — or to flip, stretch and tease apart loopy coils of bowel.

But most doctors aren't superstars (at least not in the minds of others). They're fairly bright and possess adequate manual skills.

People believe you need great hands to be a surgeon. For routine procedures like gallbladder, breast and hernia surgeries, it's not true. In reality, constant practice and repetition — holding the knife, cutting and tying vessels over and over again — train a surgeon to do the job safely. Even those with average to below-average dexterity can go on to become experts in their fields.

In anesthesia, repetition and practice are also important, but there is less emphasis on manual skills — except when it comes to insertion of breathing tubes, nerve blocks, epidurals and heart monitors. Experience teaches the anesthetist how to best protect the body from the stresses of surgery — making sure that the brain, heart, lung and kidney are oxygenated, that blood is replaced, that body temperature is maintained and that the patient wakes up pain-free and comfortable.

To perform routine operations safely and competently, experience is far more important than innate talent.

Practice Makes Perfect

It is through the stress and humiliation of experience that we learn. The first patients I anesthetised were healthy people going for small routine operations. Everything initially went according to plan, and I had the mistaken impression it was all too easy. This did not go unnoticed by the professors, who were fully aware of my budding cockiness.

"You can put the next patient to sleep. I'll step back and you can do the whole anesthetic."

"Wow, this is great," I naïvely thought.

It was not a pretty anesthetic as far as technical proficiency was concerned. Mrs. Viola needed a hysterectomy. She was a 275-pound diabetic patient who obviously loved pasta. She had asthma, high blood pressure and very thick rolls of fat covering her stubby arms. After I attempted to start an intravenous eight times — prompting her to cry out with teary eyes, in front of everyone, "Why you hurt me so much! You not know how to do it?" — I was finally able to anesthetise her.

However, this was only after she had turned various shades of blue as I struggled to deliver oxygen into her lungs; the surgeon screamed at me numerous times for not giving enough muscle-paralysis drugs; and her blood pressure jumped so wildly up and down that the anesthetic record of it resembled the spiked teeth of a large saw.

I anxiously waited for her to awake and respond after the surgery, fearing that she had suffered a stroke or heart attack because of my anesthetic. When she eventually awoke in the recovery room, I silently thanked God for the tremendous resilience of the human body.

After this sweat-soaked, panic-stricken nightmare of an anesthetic, I was chastened back to humility. But the experience was a wonderful lesson. With the subsequent variants of patients like Mrs. Viola, I was prepared and ready.

You might wonder whether recently graduated surgeons have had enough experience to operate without supervision. In every operative specialty, there are those who don't have natural technical abilities but will try to improve. They will seek as much clinical experience as possible, beg to have more time in the operating room and want to perform the entire procedure themselves. These are the people you want around you during an operation.

However, some residents aren't aggressive and show less enthusiasm. They may have below-average technical skills. Because of this, the professors have less confidence in them and will not let them perform more dangerous and complex procedures. Because they are passive, these residents don't try to gain extra experience. They don't push for more operating-room time. This cycle continues throughout the residency. Upon graduation, they have minimal or inadequate experience. These are the people you do not want to have in the operating room.

A colleague from medical school was accepted into a tough surgical program. He was a pleasant fellow but perhaps a bit too nice — I was actually surprised he was accepted into this surgical program that had a reputation for chewing graduates up and spitting them out. News of his travails filtered back to us. He started off badly by not asserting and defending his opinions or answers. When he answered questions, his demeanor was not strong. Senior staff thought he was weak or incompetent. Unfortunately, he didn't aggressively push back — he needed to prove to others they were wrong. He lost confidence, which made others stop challenging him. Eventually, he was let go from the program.

I felt sorry for him. Had the senior professors been more supportive or patient with him, he might have eventually blossomed, seizing the opportunities to improve his skills and gain confidence. Was it unfair? Many would say so. But many surgical programs assume the student is aggressive and wants to learn — changing attitudes is not their responsibility. They believe the program functions only to provide ample challenge and clinical experience.

In any program, experience not only hones technical skills, but helps to develop the ability to avoid and recognize mistakes. During training, you're repeatedly told that mistakes will inevitably occur.

A good clinician is aware of the complications that can occur with each procedure. Being aware is important. When recognizing a mistake, he or she knows the best way to fix it. Given that more than half of hospital mistakes occur in the surgical service, with most of these errors taking place in the operating room, it's an important issue.

Studies have shown that experience is an important factor related to better operating room safety. J.D. Birkmeyer et al., showed this in an analysis of 474,108 procedures published in the *New England Journal of Medicine*. The more often a doctor has performed a certain procedure, the less likely it is that the patient will die.

In a hospital study, the *Canadian Institute of Health Information* analyzed over 180,000 procedures and found that the hospitals that performed the highest volume of procedures — like lobectomy (removal of certain parts of the lungs) or carotid endarterectomy (cleaning out blockages of neck vessels to prevent strokes) — have lower death rates than low-volume hospitals. This is probably an indication that practice does make perfect, not just for the surgeon, but for the entire O.R. team, especially for these larger, more complex procedures.

Lack of experience is the likely explanation for the "first year curse." I've observed the inevitable complications and mini-disasters that occur in the *first year* of solo practice. Despite rigorous training, there will always be something you have read about but have personally never encountered. In fact, most O.R. doctors will say they were not completely comfortable and confident in the operating room until the first year had passed. So, it is experience that determines success or failure — which can mean life or death — during an operation. My next examples illustrate this.

The Temp

I liked Dr. Bach from the first time I met him. He wore large dark-rimmed glasses and his boyish face was full of friendly enthusiasm. He was obviously energized by his love of surgery and the excitement of being the surgeon on call. But what I really admired about him was his straightforward, non-arrogant attitude.

He was the "locum" surgeon. A locum doctor is a short-term replacement who fills in for established doctors who are on vacation. It's an opportunity for graduates who have not yet obtained a permanent position to earn extra income and also gain some "real world" experience and make decisions independently without the constant supervision of a teaching hospital.

He was hunched over the sleeping patient's splayed grey guts — all 25 feet of large and small intestine — as they lay coiled, moist and contracting over the surgical field. Sweat beaded on his forehead as he desperately examined small sections, looking for a telltale sign. Somewhere in the tangled mess there was a small hole in the gut wall, which was causing fever, a rigid, painful abdomen and the leaking "air sign" seen on x-ray. And yet he could not find the hole, even after six methodical, section-by-section examinations of the entire area.

After over an hour of fruitless searching, he suddenly looked up at us and said, "Call Dr. Hagen, please."

Dr. Hagen is the chief of surgery. An athletic man with piercing blue eyes and a presence that radiates energy and action, you feel that he is always ready to vigorously pounce at a problem. A slick veteran surgeon, he is also one of the nicest people to work with. Even if it was the middle of the night, if Dr. Hagen was available, he would come in — without protest or profanity — because he always tries to help his colleagues.

After waiting another 20 minutes, Dr. Hagen bounded in with a "Hello" and a "What seems to be the problem?"

After scrubbing and getting his surgical greens and gloves on, he took over from Dr. Bach and stood beside the patient. Within seconds, his hands dug deep within the abdominal cavity, reached in to pull out a huge coiled mass of intestines that he set out to one side of the body. A few minutes later, probing and feeling within the patient, he casually said, "Here it is."

"You've got to move the entire gut to one side like this," he explained to Dr. Bach, "to clear the site, and usually start to look here."

After Dr. Hagen departed, Dr. Bach looked at us and said, "He's got a lot more experience than I have."

Despite the difficulty Dr. Bach experienced, I admired him. He tried his best for this patient and, discovering his limitations, had the wisdom to ask for help and the honesty to admit he needed it.

Return to Tiger Country

Even talented surgeons like Dr. Huynh learn the value of experience in life or death situations.

While on emergency call as chief resident, he explained how he and another resident were trying to stop massive bleeding from a duodenal ulcer. With the patient cut open, blood rapidly filling the abdominal cavity and the blood pressure falling, they desperately searched for the blood-spewing hole in the duodenum — a part of the gut that connects to the stomach. Their plan was to find the ulcer and the pumping artery within it and do a "plug the dyke" maneuver — plug it up with a finger while sewing around it. But the gut was too swollen and thickened and the welling blood made it impossible to find the hole.

Dr. Bryce Taylor, the staff person, came in and repeatedly questioned them about their plan to stop the bleeding.

Finally, he asked, "What is the blood supply to this part of the duodenum?" Taylor then calmly reached into the bloodied abdominal cavity and within seconds, produced a throbbing vessel, pinched between his fingers.

"The gastro-duodenal artery. Here, clamp this." And with that, the bleeding stopped.

Overtime

Contributing further to reduced clinical experience are the limitations in resident work hours for operating room and emergency call that have been in place over the last five years.

No one would argue that too much emergency call and hospital work in the past resulted in residents who were exhausted, unsafe, stressed and depressed. Rules restricting hospital work hours have resulted in happier, more satisfied trainees, and have significantly decreased the number of doctors who quit. The problem now is the potentially severe decrease in vital clinical experience during training.

A recent surgical journal measured a 50 to 70 percent decrease in the number of operations experienced by junior residents compared to the years before the limitation imposed on resident work hours. Other studies have noted a 40 percent decrease in the number of advanced and basic surgical procedures senior residents experience. Only 18 percent of residents polled in one study believed their training adequately prepared them for advanced surgical procedures.

Speaking to some recently graduated surgeons, as well as those who graduated five or six years ago, there is general agreement that the responsibilities of a senior surgical resident have decreased over the last few years. In the past, a senior resident would do most of a major operation, and be classified an "independent operator." The staff person would stand completely back or not even be present in the operating room. There was consensus that at the senior resident level they could competently perform major operations, having been involved with similar operations in the past.

The recent drop in senior resident experience has important consequences. First, many of the senior residents aren't confident flying solo, so the staff persons supervise closely, leaving less opportunity for a senior resident to operate from start to finish by themselves. Given the medical–legal climate that exists today, supervisors closely lord over these inexperienced residents, keenly aware that the ultimate responsibility for patient safety rests with them.

It can be a frightening experience for the rest of us in the O.R. when some inexperienced, recently graduated doctors don't know their limitations.

Like the Harvard-trained and recently graduated orthopedics locum who took four hours to fix a fractured hip — normally a 60-minute case. For some odd reason, in order to view the fracture site, he repeatedly insisted on rotating the patient on the operating table, rather than just rotating the mobile C-arm on the portable x-ray machine. Everyone in the operating room could sense his insecurity and inexperience. The prolonged surgical time meant more blood loss, struggles to keep the patient warm and, of course, agony for everyone else in the O.R. as we suffered with the surgeon's indecision and uncertainty.

Another time, we expected a newly graduated locum surgeon to easily remove a "hot" infected gallbladder during emergency surgery.

The gallbladder looks like a small inflated balloon attached under the edge of the liver. After clipping the artery and duct at the neck of the balloon, the gallbladder is teased and dissected off the lower liver — akin to gently peeling the balloon off the liver — and then removed as a whole from the body.

We watched in horror as this surgeon awkwardly fumbled with the equipment and then repeatedly tore small, bloody, chewed-up bits of the gallbladder out of the patient. It was an oozing, bloody mess in the end.

When confronted by this inexperience, the rest of us in the O.R. try to make indirect comments about competency — "Boy, there's a lot of bleeding. . . . Do you think we're going to need blood? . . . What about another approach?" Or finally, "Do you want us to call the other staff person?"

It's those who don't ask for assistance that scare us.

Performance Anxiety

Yet, I must admit, I have sympathy for newly graduated doctors, who practice solo for the first time. The sudden realization that a teaching staff person is not nearby can be a very daunting experience. During the years of training, the reassuring presence of a staff person reduces anxiety. Clinical problems can be discussed with another doctor, and when the proverbial crap hits the fan, another set of hands is most useful.

I recall my first day as a staff anesthetist at my hospital. I was called to work a day earlier than scheduled — the day I had planned not to work, but to just familiarize myself with the O.R.

Not all O.R.s are the same. There can be five or six manufacturers for every piece of operating room equipment — with each device having slightly different operating characteristics. You've got to familiarize yourself with the idiosyncrasies of the equipment. And even locating where instruments, drugs and fluids are located can be frustrating. (It's difficult enough to find which floor the operating room is on and where the washrooms are.)

I rushed in to the hospital that day, with sympathetic nurses pointing me in the general direction of the operating rooms. After struggling into O.R. greens, I dashed out to the O.R. desk and discovered to my relief that the first case was a routine varicose vein operation. The stars, it seemed, were in my favor, for the patient was young and healthy.

I went to see her in the pre-surgical area. She was a striking blonde-haired woman in her early 40s, sitting in a regal manner with her back straight and in firm contact with the support of the chair. She sternly regarded me as I approached her.

"Hello," I said as I smiled and tried to convey the air of a calm and cool veteran — someone who had seen it all, who would regard giving anesthetic for such a simple operation to be as routine as clipping fingernails.

"I'm giving you your anesthesia today."

She focused on me with steel-blue eyes and a face that registered not a sliver of warmth. Before I could say anything more, she began speaking in the manner of a judge reading the rules of the court. "My name is Sally Leslie. I'm one of the top medical litigation lawyers in the city. I have reviewed the records of this hospital, of its surgeons and employees. I've looked at the number of complaints and malpractice decisions, and I've found the rates here to be the lowest of all the hospitals. And so I have come here for my surgery."

I was momentarily speechless, but I recovered and completed my preoperative assessment. In a state of anxiety and fear, I hurried out to prepare for the operation.

In the operating room, I discovered to my horror that the anesthetic machine was an older model that I was unfamiliar with. Having trained with modern machines, the gauges, dials and tubing of this device looked like a Rube Goldberg–version of the normal machine. I quickly reviewed the important details — oxygen source, flush valve, fresh gas supplies, ventilator, suction and — especially after my confidence-sapping introduction to Ms. Leslie — the emergency resuscitation drugs.

I would've definitely appreciated another ten minutes to carefully examine the set up. But suddenly, the operating room door flew open and in strode Ms. Leslie. She marched to the operating table and lay down. At this point, I felt like shrieking at everyone, "Get out of the room now and go back. I really don't feel ready to start this anesthetic." But it was too late. Somehow, I knew that a remark like that would not engender much confidence in me from anyone.

When you begin practice in the O.R., all eyes focus upon you. The nurses, assistant and surgeon stand by the patient as you begin your anesthetic. At that moment, you feel as though you're onstage. Don't let your hands shake! You're silently evaluated by the veterans surrounding you: Is he confident, or full of fear? Does he have good technical skills? Does he look like he's had lots of experience? Does he know what he's doing?

With great effort, I struggled to minimize the trembling of my hands, and somehow started the intravenous. As I was about to inject the first dose, Ms. Leslie glared up at me. In a quiet, sinister voice that nearly froze my blood she whispered, "You better do a good job."

A terrible smile accompanied that statement.

In the end, the anesthetic and surgery were uncomplicated. I transferred her, with much relief, into the recovery room. But I'll admit, it wasn't one of my best anesthetics. She woke up cold and shivering. Despite the fact that I gave her anti-nausea medicines, she threw up all over the bed. And because I really wanted to avoid narcotic overdose that might lead to a respiratory arrest — just *one* of my imagined worst-case scenarios — she woke with significant soreness.

Later, I went in to the recovery room to see her and she looked like hell. She lay in her recovery room bed, shivering, groggy and injected with pain-control medicines. After having the vomit wiped from her mouth, she looked at me from the corner of a bloodshot and half-open eye and said, "You did a very good job — great anesthetic, thank you." I smiled weakly and quickly scurried away.

From *Super Mario* to Super Surgeon

As the ability of doctors to competently perform routine operations is related to experience, even greater challenges await surgeons, because complex laparoscopic "keyhole" techniques are becoming more and more common. The advantages are obvious: no big ugly scar, less pain, faster recovery and a good visualization of internal body structures. But mastering this type of surgery, especially advanced surgery involving repair and removal of major and delicate organs, requires much more skill than other types of surgery do.

It's easier to train a person to become good in non-laparoscopic open surgery. The resident can directly feel the tissue being operated on and learn its textures, strengths and properties. Also, students can observe their own hands while operating, thus allowing them to mimic the hand techniques of their teachers. In fact, the teacher will demonstrate how to hold instruments and techniques with his or her own hands and can guide the hands of the student to demonstrate an action. None of this is possible with laparoscopic surgery.

With laparoscopic techniques, the operators can't look at their own hands because their eyes are focused on the video screen. The long surgical instruments are poked from outside the patient, through the skin, with the other end inside the body, so there is a "fulcrum" effect — movement of the operator's hands from outside the body causes the instrument inside the body (seen on the video screen) to move in the opposite direction . . . the opposite of what you would intuitively expect.

Residents must also translate a two-dimensional video image into three-dimensional actions within the body. A recent study showed that avid video gamers have a significant advantage mastering the laparoscopic techniques compared to others. Also, the need to sometimes be ambidextrous is more frequent in laparoscopic operations.

Finally, operating with long instruments from outside the body means surgeons lose the ability to directly touch and feel the tissue. Instead, they learn how things resist when grasped and pulled by instruments probing within the body.

It's not surprising then that a recent study indicates that perhaps 4 percent of surgical residents will not be able to master these advanced laparoscopic surgeries.

The New Guy

The importance of experience with advanced techniques was illustrated when I observed a new senior resident, soon to graduate, trying to remove a bowel cancer laparoscopically (with keyhole surgery techniques) under the supervision of a staff person. The resident wanted to perform most of the surgery herself.

These situations present a continuing dilemma in medical education. Obviously, the patient wants a good outcome but has signed a paper authorizing the resident to assist. But, in truth, we all know that many of the surgeries, in whole or part, are actually done by the resident under supervision of the staff person. This is the way, from the very beginnings of surgical training, that doctors have been taught.

We all hope that the new resident isn't a complete dolt, and the supervision of the staff person will prevent major errors. But it's impossible for the supervision to be absolute and there are always unknowns only revealed during surgery — you don't know how much skill and understanding a resident has until they perform the operation.

During this surgery, I could see that the staff person was uncomfortable. Frequently, he would stop and suggest improvements and even take over the surgery to demonstrate. On the other hand, the senior resident kept asking to resume the procedure herself. She obviously wanted as much operating time as possible. We could all see that her technique was not as slick as a veteran's — she handled the tissue awkwardly, her tissue dissections were ragged and bloody, and her suture lines were not quite neat and pat.

There was a long hesitation after the last sewing connecting the two ends of the bowel was completed. The staff person repeatedly tested for leaks. He looked stressed. Finally he allowed the operation to finish.

Afterwards, in the locker room, I asked him about the surgery.

"Yeah, I was not 100 percent happy. She didn't dissect [tease apart tissue] as well as I would have wanted, and it was bloody. I was not really sure that all sutures [sewing threads] connected the actual bowel tissue. It was hard to see that every suture was a good one. That's why I really took time to check for leaks.

"It's not like open surgery, where my hands can show how to properly hold things and do a procedure, or even guide her hands with mine.

"But she is a senior resident. She wants the experience. I've got to help her to learn. That's my role. She could obviously do the operation, though not as perfectly as I would have liked."

He paused. "We'll just have to see."

Unfortunately, his fears were realized two days later, when the bowel did develop a leak, and the patient returned to the operating room for emergency surgery.

Virtual O.R.

Since many graduating surgical residents feel they lack the necessary experience, what can be done to solve this problem? There is a trend to enroll in fellowship, post-graduation training after having completed the normal residency training — though it must be discouraging for many, who, after completing years of arduous training, realize they have to do more.

In Europe, the level of experience upon graduation is even less. Many come to North America in order to have far more operating experience than back home.

There is even a movement at some schools in North America to increase the length of undergraduate residency training.

But more and more, the use of surgical simulators, as well as anesthesia simulators, is increasing, with the hope that they will accelerate learning by replacing the missing operating-room experience. Just as virtual simulators are commonplace in aviation training, the concept can be adapted for surgical and anesthesia training.

These complex machines allow the student to perform a simulated operation with lifelike images, realistic interactions between organs and instruments — an organ will deform when pressed or an object will fall on the screen when dropped — along with realistic reactions, like bleeding or leaking.

The most sophisticated machines even have sensory feedback relayed through the instruments to simulate the experience of moving, grabbing, pulling and cutting tissue.

Most residents love the simulators. They can practice and not harm patients. Some feel that not worrying about this helps them to concentrate and in this way learn faster.

Some studies have shown significant improvement in performance after using simulators, with shorter operating times and fewer errors compared to those who did not. Other studies revealed mixed results, showing no reliable difference between those trained with the aid of a simulator compared to those trained with real patients.

As of now, the use of simulators is not widespread, but it is increasing. Cost is a big issue. But if operative experience on real patients has decreased and the benefit of simulators can be proven, these machines will be routinely used in the future.

School's Out?

Let's now explore the competency of doctors at different types of hospitals. Most people believe that academic expertise at university teaching hospitals leads to lower operative deaths than at non-teaching hospitals. Also, the most complex procedures, like liver transplants and specialized brain operations, can only be done at large university centers.

For routine procedures done at either teaching or non-teaching hospitals, studies have shown no difference in the number of deaths after operations, either in the short- or long-term.

As mentioned before, a patient's anesthetic and surgery carried out at a teaching hospital will be done in part by a student with limited experience. Mistakes will be made and corrected. Some learning will occur during the operation.

There is the incorrect belief that an operating room doctor at a university hospital is more skilled than a doctor in a community, non-teaching hospital. This is not always the case. There are many academic surgeons and anesthetists who have wonderful skills, but one shouldn't assume there aren't community doctors who are better. The volume of routine cases performed at a teaching hospital can be much lower than at a busy community hospital. And if the residents perform many of the procedures, the staff person has less total operating experience.

To illustrate, let me compare a radical prostate operation performed at a community hospital to one performed at a university hospital. At the teaching hospital, the senior resident performs most of the operation with the staff person occasionally taking over. Progress is much slower, resulting in a three- to four-hour operation, and the operative field is bloodier, requiring perhaps two to five units of transfused blood. In contrast, at the community hospital, two veteran urologists (who probably have each performed three times the number of prostate operations as a university urologist) work in tandem. The result is a one-and-a-half-hour operation with little or no blood transfused. (In fact, it's not uncommon for young anesthetists starting at community hospitals to overestimate the length of surgery and, having just given another hour's worth of paralyzing-drugs, are shocked when the surgeon says, "We'll be done in ten minutes." It happened numerous times when I began.)

Is the length of the surgery and the amount of transfused blood a concern? There is evidence that blood given during an operation permanently modifies the immune system. With each unit of blood the risk of postoperative infection increases. The risk of cancer recurrence may also be higher when more than two units of blood are given. The longer the surgery and the longer the patient is exposed to anesthetic agents, the greater the stress to the body.

Judgment Day

I've discussed the importance of experience in a good operating room doctor. But even the most promising career in the operating room can be destroyed by bad judgment. I'm not writing about incompetent doctors who should not have graduated from medical school in the first place. Instead, these are people who started with all the tools for success — intelligence, technical skills, people skills — yet cracked after their careers began to flourish.

The common factors in these cases are an overwhelming practice, then stress and, finally, depression and the inability to cope with work.

Dr. Dryden was a case in point. In his mid-30s, thin and tall, with a dark complexion, relaxed expression and soft voice, he had no trouble filling his office with patients. An obstetric graduate of the North American system as well as the English one, his qualifications and experience were impressive.

He began his practice at about the same time I did. I can remember talking with him about our careers. It seemed that he would have a fulfilling and successful future.

From the start, he was in high demand. He had privileges at not one but two hospitals. His operating-room lists were full of cases. Any person working with him knew that it would be a very busy day. Pages, calls and trips to the delivery ward would interrupt the day — consults to see, confirmation of bookings and requests for his immediate presence at the delivery of a baby. In the chaos of it all, it seemed that he was doing well.

But after about three years, rumors were starting to spread — whispers about high complication rates during surgery and difficulty reaching him when there were problems. He always seemed to be on the run, going from one case to another and even one hospital to another, then back again.

Eventually, due to accumulating complaints and serious

incidents, one hospital suspended him.

The final cases before his suspension are good examples of poor judgment. In the first case, he could not be contacted when his elderly patient, who had a hysterectomy, was dying of postoperative infection and organ failure in the intensive care unit. The decision to do the surgery in the first place was questionable. Though there had been some scant bleeding from her uterus, all tests had ruled out cancer. There was no urgency to do any surgery. She was 87 years old with a long history of heart disease, diabetes and high blood pressure. In other words, she was a very poor surgical candidate, with a high risk of postoperative complications. The patient insisted on an operation. Dr. Dryden did little to dissuade her and instead went ahead.

In his final case, another obstetrician on call told the O.R. to get ready to do an emergency C-section. He warned that fetal heart tracing was decelerating, indicating that the baby was not getting enough oxygen in the womb. Dr. Dryden was paged, and when he eventually called back, he insisted that everyone wait until he arrived so he could perform the surgery. The staff rushed and prepared in the operating room, with the mother draped and ready for the incision. The monitored sounds of the baby's declining heart beeped ominously while the gowned and gloved doctors and nurses waited silently and listened in agony. After at least ten minutes, the obstetrician on call couldn't wait a minute more.

Nothing can adequately describe the horror of seeing the pale, limp body as it was handed from the womb for resuscitation, or the anger of the people in the O.R. as Dr. Dryden arrived at this point and asked why they had started without him.

He made these terrible medical decisions that harmed his patients. However, they were not the true measure of the man before his erratic behavior began — a person who was genuinely concerned about his patients' welfare. True, it was unforgiveable to work so hard in the pursuit of recognition and perhaps monetary gain. But once he started the cycle of overwork, the constant stress blinded him to the dangers it created and eventually led to a serious major depression — one that caused him to lose sight of the common sense of patient care. At his discipline hearing, he broke down and admitted his faults.

Every doctor has a limit to the amount of job-induced stress they can take. Some can thrive under intense conditions — others must find escape from the pressure to find balance. The final measure of competent doctors is their awareness of their own limitations.

CHAPTER 5

Outside of the O.R.

There are places in the hospital that don't have the excitement or drama of the emergency and operating rooms. Yet, these less hectic areas — administration, cafeteria, physiotherapy and dietary departments; the basement; the autopsy room and the morgue — each offer a unique perspective on the hospital.

Administration

I've got to admit that running a hospital is difficult job. Each year, as our population ages, the demand for hospital services steadily increases. Yet, the hospital is expected to meet this increase while struggling with decreasing funds. On the other hand, many of us who work in hospital have become cynical about the administration; we've become disillusioned by poor decisions and a lack of consultation.

The CEO is, of course, the leader of the hospital. He or she was chosen after an arduous selection process. The winning candidate was supposed to have the vision, communication skills and financial expertise to deliver leading-edge services to the community. For many the CEO was looked at as a champion who would rescue the hospital from crisis.

In reality, most CEOs fear their jobs will be taken over by government supervisors if budgets aren't kept in line. This potential exists wherever government is involved in running a national health service: for example, England, Australia and Canada. Thus, the Chosen One ends up becoming a bean counter — slashing programs to the bone and decreasing services while hanging onto his job.

This creates tremendous friction between the medical staff and administration as the doctors and nurses find valuable programs reduced or eliminated in cost-saving measures: gone are post–heart attack rehab programs (which have been proven to decrease the chance of repeat heart attacks) and diabetic management programs (that reduce kidney disease and amputation rates in patients). These are examples of effective programs that can get axed.

At many hospitals across the country, disagreements between the doctors and the CEO can reach a boiling point. As a result, ad hoc medical groups meet in secrecy, where staff members scream in rebellion, raise their fists and vent their spleens. Emboldened by the pack mentality and their own frustration, the doctors make the ultimate call: let's fire and replace the CEO.

However, in most cases, the results are predictable; nothing happens and the CEO carries on. Why? The truth is, we doctors think we're smart enough to fight a CEO, when in fact, we're not. We're just babes in the woods, sacrificial lambs, girl and boy scouts — think of any overused metaphor describing inexperienced naïfs confronting a seasoned business executive, and it applies.

The reasons we're frequently unsuccessful fighting administration are simple. We have worked hard to be accepted into medical schools. We then immerse ourselves in study, absorbing mountains of medical information. This leaves little time to learn important skills in the non-clinical world; doctors can gather evidence about a disease, but we don't know how to gather evidence about administrative matters; we know the protocols to fight illness with drugs and surgery, yet are ignorant about strategies to raise funds, garner public support and draw media attention to hospital problems or successes.

Additionally, given that we are caregivers, most doctors have a trusting nature. And in a clinical setting, the people we deal with are, for the most part, decent and helpful.

However, outside the clinical setting, people aren't always so nice. We've never learned to cultivate powerful allies, get outsiders' help, identify and handle those who would mislead or deceive us — we've had no lessons on how to be a bit of a hard ass. It's no wonder that most physicians are conned easily, tend to make terrible investors and are bad at business.

Finally, some doctors develop the attitude that they are special after dealing with life-and-death issues, and so become self-important fools doomed to political failure in the non-clinical world.

The CEO gives the approval for major decisions and he or she is ultimately responsible for the overall performance of the hospital. However, the quality of each clinical service in hospital — such as surgical, maternity or geriatric — is directly related to the competency of individual program directors. It's obvious when leaders of specific programs don't have a firm grasp on problems or are unable to find solutions. Their questionable decisions are a wonderful source of humorous stories.

Unfortunately, the inability of many administrators and program directors to solve problems is quite pervasive across the whole managed-care system. And even if an incompetent administrator loses his or her job, they magically pop up at another hospital. It's like a perpetual employment game of health musical chairs where everyone rotates to the next job until the music inevitably stops again.

Despite budgetary restraints, I've observed renovations to the administrative offices, creating space to accommodate more administrative assistants in the growing bureaucracy. Their spacious offices are outfitted with fine accoutrements — sturdy desks, comfortable Herman Miller chairs in the conference room, relaxing artwork and tastefully decorated walls.

We contrast this with the clinical staff's lounges and meeting rooms, which are cramped and dimly lit, and furnished with bargain chairs and sofas set on 1980s-era grey-green carpeting. Another dreary cubbyhole is the call room, where staff can rest overnight. Despite numerous complaints, it's located in the basement, two distant floors from the operating rooms. Small and dark, it's been used numerous times by other employees for late-night rendezvous. Even more irritating is that the house-keeping staff insist on cleaning the room — though the bed sheets aren't changed — at midnight, when doctors are trying to sleep. Despite numerous e-mails, letters and complaints, nothing changes.

Intentionally or not, they're giving us a message: the bureaucrats require quality surroundings. The clinicians and non-bureaucrats get the leftovers.

In the hospital, most problems involve financial and staffing issues. When the administration is confronted with problems too difficult to handle, consultants are hired. Consultants charge $1,500 to $2,000 per day. For prices like this, you might expect some useful solutions. Unfortunately, their recommendations are unimpressive. When these consultants complete their reports and are paid their enormous fees, it seems only *their* fiscal situation has significantly improved.

We've already had a consultant investigate operational efficiencies (cost savings) in the O.R. She was a pleasant woman — full of smiles, though not very communicative. She also did not seem to know her way around the operating rooms. This was a strange deficit considering her role was to help the operating room run smoothly. She didn't want to enter the operating rooms, preferring to stand outside each room and observe through the window. Unsurprisingly, her report had less value than the paper it was printed upon.

On another occasion, a consultant was asked to unify departments after two hospitals had merged. Just as two companies can have problems integrating staff, so too can merging hospitals. After weeks of interviews with members of all departments, everyone looked forward to the solutions. The final report was issued. In it, the consultant suggested we carry on best we could and keep trying; essentially, he told us: good luck. Years later, people within many departments are still bickering with each other.

As mentioned before, when decisions are made by the administration, they're frequently done without consultation with those most affected. A perfect example is the time we came to work and found the operating room thermostats, which used to be at shoulder height, had been moved to seven-and-a-half feet up on the wall.

Temperature regulation is not an insignificant issue in the operating room. Equipment must be kept at a certain temperature to avoid condensation and malfunction. Sometimes the room has to be very warm for the patient. Other times the temperature has to be decreased to accommodate the surgeon who must stand for hours during a difficult case. Whatever the reason, frequent temperature adjustments occur. The personnel in the operating room must be in full control of temperature changes and be available at a moment's notice to adjust the thermostat. You can imagine how awkward it would be for someone to balance on a stool to try to read and adjust a thermostat that's seven-and-a-half feet up on the wall.

I phoned down to administration and talked to the vice president of operations, Brenda.

"Hi Brenda. We're all kind of shocked to see that the thermostats are seven-and-a-half feet up on the wall. It's very difficult for us to change the temperature in the room. Why has this been done?"

There was some agitation in her voice when she replied. "Thermostats have been frequently broken and we think the shoulders of people rubbing against them is causing this problem. So we repositioned them."

In fact, the thermostats had been dismantled by operating room staff who tried to fix them. Our frequent complaints about malfunctioning thermostats were ignored. Damage to thermostats was not the problem; they just weren't working well. We were trying to fix the problem ourselves.

"I was a nurse once you know," she continued. "I'm not that tall. Nurses in the operating room should be able to stand on a stool all day." And then she hung up.

That is why our hospital, somewhat proudly, has the highest operating room thermostats in North America — and probably the world.

A situation like this allows us to laugh at ourselves. Unfortunately, many people in administration lack any sense of humor. Having a sense of humor is vital in a stress-filled hospital. When used properly, it makes others feel better; it diffuses tense situations, and keeps people grounded. For those in administration, humorous criticism is a personal affront, and the ability to admit errors is impossible.

A little while ago, a senior administrator approached me before a meeting. In the preceding months, the hospital had been through a rash of bad publicity and negative reports.

"Paul, I just want to tell you this ship had been going in the wrong direction. It's been turned around and now the ship is pointed in the right direction," she said with earnest enthusiasm in her eyes.

In my mind, a picture of the RMS *Titanic* heading towards the glacier flashed momentarily.

Not wishing to miss an opportunity at a humorous dig and assuming she could take some gentle ribbing, I replied, "But Christine, weren't you on deck when the ship was heading in the wrong direction?"

Unfortunately, all she did was look at me in distress, then turn around.

It's not just the bad decisions that are frustrating. Even when requests are made to address important issues, they're ignored. Sometimes, if a routine problem is ignored long enough, it can become a huge, embarrassing event.

During a long, hot summer, when the air-conditioning was not working, the urinal in the male washroom located beside the change room stopped flushing. After a number of people had used it, tried to flush and failed, a formal requisition was sent for repair. In the interim, the reservoir was doused frequently with disinfectants. However, robust bacteria combined with the hot, humid conditions created a greenish-yellow stagnating collection in the basin. It released a distinctive terrible smell into the entire locker room. After many days, despite frequent requests, the problem was not addressed.

In the movie *Apocalypse Now*, the eccentric Lt. Colonel Kilgore flies through a misty, dangerous battle zone, sniffs the air and declares, "I love the smell of napalm in the morning." When we arrived into the change room every morning, for the next two weeks, the smell was so overpowering, it was like entering a battle zone. Perhaps only deranged people like Lt. Colonel Kilgore and hospital staff could continue to work under conditions like these.

Seriously, it really wasn't a great way to start the day. With only a single flush toilet to use as the alternative, and with a busy operating room leaving little time for private business between cases, staff had to frequently run out into the hallway for the public washrooms — and face lineups there. (Privately, semi-serious discussions were made about urinating into the sink. However, even in our desperate state, we felt decorum would suffer. The idea was abandoned.)

I recall trying to get the attention of a colleague, Dr. Connie, as he raced out in panic. "No time now. Must go pee before case starts," he panted as he flew by me, down to the outside washroom.

Eventually, we insisted that one of the administrators come into the washroom. I watched as she entered the change room, sniffed and stifled a gag reflex.

The next day the urinal was fixed.

The Cafeteria

Those of us who work in hospitals have a recurring dream. In this wonderful fantasy, the staff is energized during long and tiring shifts by good-tasting and nutritious cafeteria food — food that is available anytime we're free. We feel comforted, knowing the administration provides this food because they actually care about us.

Getting back to reality, when you enter the real cafeteria, you're greeted by educational materials that laud the benefits of healthy eating. They're the usual photographs of beautiful fruits and vegetables in combination with breads and meats that are part of a balanced diet.

However, there's a stark contrast between these images and the *actual* offerings. The stainless steel warmers hold sausages floating in pools of grease and a deep-fried assortment of chicken wings, nuggets, french fries and battered fish. The steamed vegetables, after having been heated for hours, are almost totally devoid of food value, reduced to nutrient-drained filler. Of course, there's delicious, watery and discolored mac and cheese. In the soup selection, you'll see offerings so loaded with sodium that you could exceed a week's dietary recommendation in a single serving.

It's at least reassuring to know that when you have your heart attack, the emergency rooms are nearby. Think positively we tell ourselves; thank God this cafeteria is located in a hospital.

Even attempts at more healthy food combinations are disappointing. What's called beef stir fry, for example, features eraser-like, chewy mystery meat. Depending on the time of day, because supplies are limited, there may not be much choice of pre-wrapped salads. Towards the end of the week, a greater number of mixed browns are available.

The real message on the nutrition posters greeting you should read, "What does not kill you will make you stronger. Bon appétit."

It wasn't always this way. Before the mantra of cost reduction at any cost, there was care in the preparation of food. Even people from outside the hospital — students and others who just wanted a good meal at a reasonable price — lined up. I suspect the hospitals were even making a small profit. When food is good and inexpensive, they will come. Now the only people who use the cafeteria are those who have no other choice. I suspect that the cafeteria will eventually be replaced with an automatic vending machine, providing packets of stale food.

It's not just the quality of food that's a problem. On certain weekends the cafeteria closes early, so those working late must fend for themselves. Alternate food vendors in other areas of the hospital run out of supplies by mid-afternoon. It's not uncommon to see crowds of relatives and visitors in the hospital wandering about in search of any available food.

I have to confess, on occasions when food was not available, I've gone looking for food in the delivery suite and on the medical wards. Essentially, I'd look for patients who were not hungry and had mistakenly been ordered suppers. I relied upon the kindness of nurses to help me obtain food.

"The lady in bed four has just delivered, is feeling sleepy and doesn't feel like eating. You can have her meal."

"Your kindness and generosity for the desperate and hungry like me will be rewarded in heaven. *God bless us every one!*" I replied, in my best Tiny Tim impression.

Once, our frustrations reached a boiling point when three staff members, including me, were on a long and arduous shift and had to abandon our "low-sodium" lunches from the cafeteria, after finding the salt levels far too high. We could not finish our meals. Later, we wandered to the cafeteria in search of food at supper time and found the doors shut. The food at the snack bars was already gone. Our hunger, combined with fatigue and disappointment, fueled our anger.

I sent a letter to the vice president of operations. In it, I quoted Napoleon Bonaparte — "An army marches on its stomach." He was one of the first generals to recognize providing good food results in energetic, motivated and satisfied troops. I gave details about the poor food quality and its lack of availability. I concluded the letter with "Where is the love?"

In response, I received a letter from a representative from the food services company supplying the hospital. Some select quotes include:

"He says the low-salt selection was overloaded with sodium. Our food is tailored to the needs of low-sodium patients. I think he must be in error." (I guess this is why all three of us gagged with the first mouthful of the chicken casserole, and then had to gulp cups of water afterwards. Could we have all had a simultaneous salty food hallucination? Unlikely.)

"Our food is of the highest standards, and we ensure that only the best is available for your cafeteria." (Certainly, road kill and mystery meats may be fresh, but do they classify as highest standards?)

"There have never been complaints about the food or food service at this cafeteria. This indicates the quality of food has never been an issue." (I suspect the people who had bad experiences have decided not to write anything, knowing that nothing would ever change; never bothered to return to the cafeteria again; or died from salt overload — so are understandably unable to write a proper letter of complaint.)

We waited. Of course, nothing changed. In my last letter to the vice president of operations, I sadly concluded with "Brenda, I'm not feeling the love."

Within the operating room, numerous jokes about the food are common. It's a little "tasteless" humor, but in this setting, it's appropriate. For example, whenever we have amputated limbs or fingers, which we must dispose of, we warn the porter to avoid the cafeteria — fearing that some of these parts might end up in the food. Could they be added to the soup to give a little extra flavor? That *je ne sais quoi* others have tasted? Just what *are* those chewy bits in the beef stir-fry? Wait a minute: doesn't the gravy look like the same substance that was spewing out of that infected gallbladder?

There is a silver lining: the food might be the greatest encouragement for patients visiting the cafeteria to recover as quickly as possible and leave the hospital.

The Physiotherapy and Dietary Departments

Physiotherapists help patients to regain lost movement and strength due to injury or disability, to heal after orthopedic operations or to recover from strokes and other neurological maladies, and they assist those with heart and breathing problems in increasing their endurance. Most patients are grateful for their physio's expertise. Staff and patients work together to rehabilitate by using exercise equipment like bikes and treadmills, along with railings and stairs.

Another overlooked area of the hospital is the dietary department, where they understand the important nutritional needs of patients. Instead of the dreary selections seen in the cafeteria, dietitians try hard to find fresher, tastier and more nutritious alternatives from hospital suppliers for the patients. I know this from experience, having eaten the food from the wards.

In addition to the great work they do, it's important to note that both departments tend to be populated by some of the most attractive people in the hospital, people who have healthy complexions and wonderful physiques. The physiotherapists know the importance of fitness and exercise and their bodies show this. It's the same with the dieticians, who know about healthy foods and healthy living.

These are good places to observe and smile at the staff.

The Basement

The bare concrete and fluorescent-lit hospital basement differs from the bright and open hallways found above ground. Many of these subterranean passages lead to distant corners where isolated and hidden departments can be found. The lack of natural light combined with the sounds of electrical generators and hissing pipes create the impression that you're moving through a claustrophobic winding tunnel. It's easy to lose your way and become disoriented as you navigate the maze of corridors. Many people have gotten lost in the basement passageways of large downtown hospitals.

The hospital is like an organism, devouring supplies and eliminating used materials through the basement. The docking stations and gateways take in endless supplies — equipment, drugs, chemicals and food — while waste packaging, used equipment, laundry and bio-toxins are carted away by large trucks.

The environmental service, responsible for temperature and ventilation throughout the hospital, is located in the basement. The hospital takes in outside air and expels used air as it breathes. In each operating room, this enables 15 air exchanges per hour to suck away leaked anesthetic gases and airborne infections. If the system breaks down, we have to close the operating rooms.

The nervous system of the hospital — the IT department and servers — is located in the cooled and insulated confines of the underground.

The basement offers ideal storage areas in its distant and remote hallways. It is a perfect "out of sight, out of mind" depot. Unwanted, bulky equipment — like incubators, wheelchairs, stretchers and outdated electronics — accumulate here. These corridors resemble large storehouses for abandoned hospital junk, full of dusty old items too difficult to throw out, or kept as backups that are soon forgotten and never used.

When I see the workers from the basement, I wonder what it's like for them to spend most of the day working in the bowels of the hospital without windows or natural light. Do they feel different from the workers above? Do they have an "us versus them" mentality? My discussions with them confirm that they do.

The type of work above and below ground differs. Above, we interact directly with patients. Those below work without patient contact, helping the sick indirectly. We're two distinct groups, separated by environment and responsibilities, yet we share the goal of assisting those in need.

Recently built hospitals have tried to end the segregation that basement workers experience. Many departments, including IT, pathology and laboratories are now located on the ground floor of the hospital. This creates a more inclusive feel to the hospital as a whole. However, in most cases, the supply entrances, waste management and the morgue are still located below ground.

Pathology

People have a certain perception of pathologists as introverted eggheads doing nothing all day except peering into microscope slides as they reject clinical medicine and shun human contact. Some people even look down on pathologists, questioning why they decided to become doctors if they don't want to interact with patients.

In fact, pathologists are essential specialists. When pathologists study tumor specimens, they must determine whether a growth is malignant or benign. And if it is a malignant tumor, what cell type is it? The cell type determines which chemotherapy and treatments can save the patient. Essentially, the pathologists tell us the story of human illness — identifying the disease, explaining how the disease began and how it develops and predicting how it will affect the patient's future and how that future can be changed with treatment.

Even after removing a cancer, the surgeon will rely on the pathologist's tissue examination surrounding the tumor to ensure the zone is clear of cancer cells, guaranteeing all the cancer has been removed.

Pathologists have garnered both positive and negative

publicity over the years. The real-life exploits of Dr. Thomas Noguchi, a Los Angeles–based medical examiner, propelled pathology into the limelight. As chief medical examiner in Los Angeles County, he performed autopsies on the rich and famous — Marilyn Monroe, Robert F. Kennedy and John Belushi, to name just a few. He came to be known as the "coroner to the stars." Fictional medical examiners, like Kay Scarpetta in Patricia Cornwell's novels and those in the television series *CSI*, have also fascinated the public.

On the other hand, some people hold onto negative associations with the discipline, remembering the pathologist that missed the presence of cancerous cells in tissue samples that resulted in a patient's death, or a forensic pathologist's faulty conclusions that led to an innocent person being falsely imprisoned.

In the past, it was difficult to find people who wanted to become pathologists. Today, most of the residency positions are filled. There are two reasons for this reversal. First, there's the issue of lifestyle. Today, most doctors don't want a career that consumes their entire life. In pathology, the hours are 8 a.m. to 4 p.m., and there are almost no emergency calls. Second, it pays a good income from the first day of work; pathologists don't have to build a practice. That's why pathology is one of the most sought-after residency positions today.

There's a lot to learn in the residency and there are very difficult exams to pass. Though fantastic verbal skills aren't needed, excellent written skills — to be able to diagnose clearly and explain findings — are essential.

The field of pathology is divided into numerous subspecialties, such as bone pathology, neuropathology (concerning the nervous system) and other organ-specific subspecialties. Molecular pathology is a "cutting edge" subspecialty that looks deep into the cell to examine the DNA and building blocks of life in order to study disease. Forensic pathology has also been gaining attention.

The Autopsy Room

My association with Dr. Lee had previously been intermittent and distant. Though we had exchanged hellos at hospital meetings and in the cafeteria, our principal interaction was through the telephone.

When the surgeon sends a tissue sample to pathology, we wait for the analysis to be telephoned into the operating room. I usually answer the phone and then link Dr. Lee, via intercom, to the surgeon. Dr. Lee concisely defines tissue type, tissue margins and gives cogent recommendations to the surgeon, in a cool, precise, professional manner and with an accent.

When asking Dr. Lee for a tour of the pathology department and autopsy room, however, I didn't encounter an icy professional but a warm and friendly person who generously gave his time to assist me. Dr. Lee accompanied me to the autopsy room and morgue. He bemoaned the fact that fewer and fewer autopsies are being done. Today, most relatives rely on the doctor to explain the cause of death. Only when there is suspicion of a cover-up are autopsies requested by relatives. Doctors don't ask for many autopsies either. They lazily believe the high-tech diagnostic tools are all they need to pinpoint the cause of death.

However, autopsies accomplish a useful purpose. Studies show that one-third of death certificates incorrectly identify the cause of death. Half of all autopsies reveal disease findings that weren't suspected. Ten percent of unexpected findings can only be found with an autopsy.

As we proceeded into the autopsy room, located in an isolated section of the basement, Dr. Lee unlocked a thick metallic door. He revealed a room that was not built with comfort or aesthetics in mind.

A grim stainless-steel table is anchored in the middle of the cold room. The table edges have a raised border and on the surface, holes are strategically placed to catch body fluids that might ooze and drip. There are numerous grates on the floor beneath the table to facilitate drainage and cleanup after the autopsy. A blackboard inscribed with the names of organs — lungs, heart, liver — hangs from a wall. This helps the pathologist organize the autopsy and record the weights of the dissected parts.

On the opposite wall are 20 to 30 clear glass vessels displaying various organs preserved in formaldehyde. Many of these specimens have been in storage for years. The color of brains, lungs, livers and hearts fade with time — the organs develop a ghostly grey tinge from the formaldehyde. They're here for medical and legal reasons, coroner's investigations or from times when the autopsy couldn't establish cause of death. At Princeton University, parts of Einstein's brain are preserved for study, held in specimen containers like these.

While most people have their bodies buried or cremated, some choose to have their remains preserved in jars and locked in time as a memento of their lives on earth.

Most of the cutting and dissecting during autopsies is done by the anatomical pathology technologist, not the pathologist. Dr. Lee explained that many of these people are pathology residents who did not complete their exams or are foreign medical grads who could not practice medicine in North America.

I felt sympathy for the foreign doctors who are unable to practice clinical medicine. Many of them had busy practices in their native countries. Some were surgeons. It must be disappointing to end up dissecting corpses. What does a former surgeon say after returning home from the autopsy room, when his partner asks, "Did anything interesting happen at work today?"

I recall watching a technologist preparing a body for autopsy. He worked in a very businesslike way. His steady hands and deliberate incisions demonstrated skill and knowledge of human anatomy. But it also reminded me of an experienced butcher removing the best cuts of meat.

I have attended only one autopsy in my life, when I was in medical school. To say the experience was not pleasant is an understatement. I prefer interacting with living patients.

I had no problem in the dissection labs at school, studying formaldehyde-preserved specimens — the heart, the hand, the knee joint — as these were parts of bodies that didn't make me think of the whole person. But an autopsy is different. You see the entire body and it reminds you that this was recently a living, breathing person.

Researchers have discovered other factors that explain our

discomfort when we gaze at a corpse. They first asked people to consider a dead body that looks exactly like a living person. Most people were not as uncomfortable looking at this body as they were looking at an obvious corpse. The face of a corpse is distinctive: the tight facial muscles, the open mouth, the discolored lips and the unfocused eyes.

A phenomenon called the "Uncanny Valley" refers to the dip in comfort levels we feel as bodies look more and more similar to — but not identical to — a living person. If we look at a cartoon character, it can make us laugh and feel empathy towards it; we don't feel strange. However, a robot that looks almost human makes us feel uneasy. Similarly, a corpse that looks like — but isn't exactly like — a living human, makes us feel uncomfortable.

Even before the autopsy began, the smell was unpleasant. Imagine you're in a butcher shop, sniffing deeply while standing over a tray of liver, with an additional musty essence in the air.

The autopsy started with a screaming electric saw that cut through the chest bone, exposing the organs of the thorax. It was a very *Texas Chainsaw Massacre* moment. There was surprisingly little bleeding. Once the ribs were lifted away, the major organs of the thorax — the heart and lungs — were dissected and removed. Then the pathologist sliced them open and exposed their inner structures.

He discussed diseases hidden within them: he noted the plaque inside a heart vessel that had suddenly blocked blood flow, causing the yellow discoloration of dead heart muscle and he pointed out the black discoloration and destroyed tissue of "smoker's lung." The mountain of knowledge pathologists possess — the ability to give a complete story for every disease within the human body — is truly impressive and was demonstrated during the autopsy.

On the other hand, his clinical, matter-of-fact attitude, while he held a bloody organ in his hands — without unease or show of emotion — seemed bizarre to me. His level of comfort was obviously acquired after many autopsies.

I was able to tolerate the autopsy until the intestines were dissected and sliced open. There is nothing that can adequately describe the rotten, putrid smell contained within a cadaver's bowels. I found the combination of gases from rotting food and the fumes of dead intestinal cells overpowering. The odor hit me like a thick, foul wave. I felt it coat my skin and hair as it flowed over me. I imagined it would remain on my skin after the autopsy and feared others would smell it on me and turn away in disgust. The stench invaded each nostril, declaring its presence with the slightest sniff. Breathing through my mouth didn't help. All the students in the room tried to brave it out and concentrated on the pathologist, who continued to lecture without commenting about the grotesque smell. All of us were cowards. No one had the gall to exclaim — "Damn, that smells terrible!" I quietly excused myself and left.

The Morgue

Most morgues are located in the basements of hospitals. Obviously, isolating the dead from the living is a prime consideration.

Surprisingly, our present image of the morgue — a silent,

private and hidden repository for bodies after death — was not always the reality.

In 1867, Emile Zola wrote the book *Thérèse Raquin*. In it he described the Paris Morgue — a popular landmark of the city at that time, where corpses were placed in rows on concrete slabs for public viewing. Here, they presented accident and murder victims, criminals who had been executed and those who had passed away from disease or old age for all to see. Bodies were shown without regard to their state of preservation — including bodies that were already decomposed, swollen and discolored and those torn apart.

Anyone could view the bodies without restrictions based upon social status or wealth. Women in petticoats, laborers on their way home from work and children all entered this public place. The Paris Morgue was considered to be like any other popular attraction — the equivalent of a visit to the Louvre or the Eiffel Tower.

As people watched, some would joke, comment out loud or applaud the spectacle of that day.

Today, public displays of nameless corpses still attract interest. The anatomist Gunther von Hagen is the director of the Body Worlds exhibition of preserved human bodies. Through a process called plastination that removes the bodily fluids and fat and replaces them with plastic infusions, the deceased are shown in lifelike poses with bodies that have little skin, revealing the muscles and organs. Thus, the inner form, structure, mechanics and beauty of the human body are displayed. Unlike the Paris Morgue, these displays are not intended to be macabre or freakish, and there is no intended disrespect of the dead.

The hospital morgue, in contrast, upholds and maintains the dignity and solitude of the dead. Locating it in the basement, away from the public, also permits discreet transport via underground corridors, through inconspicuously marked doors, and into waiting hearses.

Dr. Lee led me to the hospital morgue. Another heavy door was unlocked and opened. We entered a temperature-controlled room filled with a few stainless steel tables. A small body wrapped in a labeled white plastic bag rested on one table. A long zipper on the bag ran from head to toe.

In city morgues, bodies are stored individually in refrigerated cabinets with temperatures approaching the freezing point. This cold preserves bodies that may lie for days until they are positively identified and examined.

At the hospital morgue, there's no need for freezing temperatures, nor are bodies individually stored. It's basically a large refrigerator storing bodies sent for autopsy or to funeral homes.

The plastic bag contained the body of a thin woman; the contours of breasts, shoulders and limbs were outlined by the bag. This was a wasted and emaciated body, and she most likely suffered from a debilitating illness like Alzheimer's disease or cancer. Death had freed her from pain.

But what was the *ultimate* cause of her death? Epidemiologists have gathered grim statistics for us: the five most frequent causes of death in hospital are heart attack, congestive heart failure (the inability of the heart to pump oxygen throughout the body), pneumonia, septicemia (blood infection) and chronic lung disease. Though this woman had a terminal condition, the ultimate cause of her death was probably due to one of these conditions.

Death in hospital can occur after a gradual deterioration, or it can occur suddenly, without warning. In cases of gradual deterioration, the patient usually experiences a series of organ failures that culminate in death.

A typical scenario is as follows: a woman is admitted with cancer that had spread into her lungs. The affected lungs can't deliver enough oxygen to the body, so the heart is stressed. The stressed heart pumps blood poorly, worsening oxygen delivery to the body. The heart can't circulate enough blood to the kidneys — kidneys that normally eliminate extra fluids — so fluid accumulates in the lungs. Finally, as the problems worsen, the heart is stressed to its limits, resulting in a heart attack and death.

The body is a finely tuned machine, where each organ system is dependent on the other systems in order to function normally. If one system starts to fail, it endangers all the other systems. The hospital staff struggles to maintain each organ system as another breaks down and must repeatedly deliver more and more bad news to the beleaguered patient and family. The end of this downward spiral is death.

On the other hand, when people in a hospital room die suddenly, it's usually due to a heart attack or a large blood clot that blocks blood circulation to the lungs. In many cases, these events occur without warning. Even if medical treatment is immediately available, in most cases it's ineffective.

Doctors and nurses will encounter patients who hover near

the line separating life and death. I don't think it helps many of us to understand the meaning of death. However, treating those who are dying does make us realize that how we die is important. We know life is finite. Animals can grieve for the dead, but there is no evidence that they, like humans, know that tomorrow may bring death. If you were to ask the general public how they would prefer to die, most would say, "In my sleep and quickly."

What is an ideal way to die? First, dying without pain and suffering is important. There are treatments that only increase distress and suffering in the last days with little chance of cure. Some patients insist on these treatments despite knowing the side effects. However, we have no right to criticize them. We can't predict how anyone will react when death stares them in the face. In David Rieff's book *Swimming in a Sea of Death: A Son's Memoir,* he describes his mother, Susan Sontag, and how she bravely fought a blood cancer when she had almost no chance of being cured. The treatments were agonizing and made her suffer horribly. Yet, she had previously overcome another cancer thought to be terminal.

In life, no one knows who will be on the "tail end" in the bell distribution — the one-in-a-million survivor who overcomes the odds. It happened to Susan Sontag before. On the other hand, I believe that most physicians wouldn't opt for treatments that have little chance of success if the treatments significantly decrease the quality of life in the last days. Doctors know the suffering this causes.

Who knows — we may be fooling ourselves. Perhaps our faith in medical statistics and outcomes prevents more doctors from occupying that "tail end" of the surviving population.

Another thing to settle before an "ideal" death is family and financial matters. Terrible stories of in-laws fighting beside the bed of a dying relative — arguing over finances and past sins — are not uncommon. It can be a horrible experience for everyone.

Thinking about death brought my thoughts back to the woman in the morgue. In my mind's eye, I can imagine her resting in a hospital bed, surrounded by family, not as a lifeless body resting on a cold table, which was my initial impression after the brief encounter in the morgue.

There are good ways to die. I hope she died peacefully, accepting her death, with the love and support of her family.

CHAPTER 6

On the Table

Details

It's natural to feel nervous if you're going to have an operation. You might even feel some panic. Knowing what to expect before and after your operation should help you relax a little more.

At our hospital, children have the opportunity to visit days before their operations. Specially trained child-care workers guide both parents and children through all aspects of the upcoming day of the operation — coming in, changing into the gown, visiting the preoperative holding area, experiencing the operating room with the anesthesia mask used for sleeping and so on. The children who have this exposure are definitely calmer and better prepared for the surgery — a benefit supported by numerous studies.

Before most operations, it's necessary to have a preoperative evaluation, which is usually done in hospital days to weeks before surgery. The medical history is reviewed and preoperative tests are performed, such as possible blood work, electrocardiogram or x-rays. All this information is collected and bundled together in preparation for the actual surgery date. Appointments with specialists may be arranged if there are important medical issues to evaluate. Finally, instructions about the operation and what to expect postoperatively are given. The date of the operation and exact time you should arrive at the hospital is confirmed.

Many of you will complain about the length of the whole process. Unless you're very lucky, accept the fact that it may be hours of questions, instructions, tests and more tests. It is a tedious process. Just make sure you pay for hours of parking time, bring a good book or your iPod, pack a snack and just try to grin and accept it. Go with the flow, and you may be one of the fortunate ones who get out early.

Try to bring any medicine you normally take at home to the preoperative evaluation, including any holistic medicines. So many times a patient forgets the name of a medication and says, "It's the yellow pill with the letter C marked on it." This is not helpful because most doctors and nurses don't identify a pill by its appearance. Make sure you can give up-to-date and accurate information about all relevant drugs and dosages.

The names of holistic medicines are important because they can cause serious problems during operations. For example, ginger, garlic, gingko and even vitamin E have been shown to increase the risk of excessive bleeding during certain surgical procedures. In general, I advise people to stop their holistic medicines at least five to seven days before a procedure involving lots of oozing or bleeding, like hip or prostate operations.

Obtaining a complete medical history is the most important part of the pre-surgical visit. It's helpful to have a paper from your family doctor summarizing your medical history and a list of medicines you are taking. Awareness of important health issues gives everyone in the O.R. a heads-up and can significantly alter surgical preparation, anesthesia technique and post-surgical care.

Interviewing patients at the clinic can be an interesting experience. Some people minimize serious medical issues or are in significant denial when questioned by someone other than their specialist or family doctor. I remember an elderly man who strenuously denied any serious health problems — which I quickly doubted when I observed his long list of drugs, his fragile appearance and, especially, the large cardiac bypass scar on his chest. Please tell us everything important during the interview.

When English is not the first language, a good interpreter is sometimes needed, though I've found relatives of patients are not always helpful.

"Now Mr. Lima, do you have any chest pain?" I ask.

The daughter interrupts. "His English is not that good. I'll speak to him for you, okay?"

"Sure, go ahead and ask him."

"Dad, do you have any chest pain?" she screams at him *in English.*

"No, I've got none," he responds in English.

She looks at me earnestly. "He says he's got no pain."

"Um, thanks."

And so it proceeds.

Why should you accept all the inconvenience of preoperative screening? Because it can save you from being canceled on the day of surgery, and sometimes it can save your life.

Here's one scenario: you're 55 years old, and you've been feeling more tired than usual. Over the last two weeks, you've had intermittent "acid" pains in the stomach. You attribute this to the repeated phone calls from your son and daughter. They are both requesting more money: your son for his partying expenses and your daughter for her upcoming wedding.

In the pre-op clinic assessment before your hernia operation, they want to do an electrocardiogram. You had one three months ago at the family doctor's and it was fine. You think it's a waste of time. The repeat cardiogram reveals big, down-spiking "Q" waves, indicating a likely heart attack that caused the sensation of gas pain and fatigue. If surgery were to proceed, research has shown a possible 37 percent chance you will have a second heart attack during or after the operation — with up to 40 percent chance of dying after this heart attack. The cardiogram? Definitely not a waste of time.

In another example, you're scheduled for a knee replacement. You're also on blood thinners for a heart condition. Because your surgeon has a very busy office, neither the surgeon nor his nurse has given you information to stop the thinners five days before the operation day. On the O.R. day, your surgery is canceled because the blood thinners increase the risk of bleeding to death during surgery. The preoperative clinic would have given you the necessary information.

The preoperative clinic will give you an outline of what to expect at each stage of the operation day. They will explain the sensations you will experience, from preparation, going under anesthetic and waking up to what to expect in terms of pain, treatment and recovery.

Studies show that only about 20 percent of important information is initially retained during this short, pre-op visit. So, two types of pamphlets are also given: one with general information about the surgical day and another with specific facts about your particular surgery.

All of this may seem like information overload. But — and this is the important point — evidence shows those receiving preoperative information and support will have significantly less postoperative pain and distress, independent of surgical or anesthetic factors. It shows that the prepared mind is a powerful factor controlling the body's response to stress, which helps to reduce suffering postoperatively.

It Pays to Complain

According to surveys, the postoperative effects that people are most concerned about are first pain, with nausea and vomiting a close second. These are not trivial issues. Both pain and feeling sick after surgery have been shown to slow overall recovery and delay a return to normal activities. Seventeen to thirty percent of patients have moderate to severe postoperative pain 24 hours after surgery. Up to 30 percent of patients suffer from post-discharge nausea 24 hours later, with about 15 percent feeling some nausea one to two days post-discharge. In one study, patients were willing to pay, on average, $100 out of pocket to avoid nausea and vomiting.

I believe all patients must speak up about pain and nausea well before the day of surgery, because effective treatments exist. If I were to have an operation, I would definitely ask, "How are you going to deal with my nausea and pain after the operation?" A good preoperative clinic, in conjunction with the anesthesia department, should have complete answers that deal with these issues and present you with their management plan.

Studies have rated various surgical procedures, predicting the degree of pain experienced upon awakening from anesthetic. Regardless of the type of surgery, younger patients experience more pain than older patients.

Low levels of pain occur after skin operations and — a surprise for most men — testicular surgery. Moderate levels of pain occur with muscle and ligament surgery, varicose-vein operations, lymph-node biopsies, thyroid, hernia and hip surgery. High levels of pain are expected with major breast operations, laparoscopic gallbladder surgery, vaginal hysterectomies, radical prostate and major gut surgery and most bone operations — especially shoulder, arm, foot, knee and spine surgery and the removal of previously inserted hardware.

Note that the ratings for the moderate and highly painful operations are based upon awakening from a standard, routine anesthetic. The good news is you needn't suffer from moderate to severe pain upon awakening if given special anti-pain medications before and after the operation and if special anesthesia techniques are used. So, if you ask about pain control and the response is "If you're sore when you wake up, we'll just inject some pain medicine," that's inadequate.

Modern postoperative pain control has undergone major advances over the last ten years. Unfortunately, allowing a person to suffer terrible pain and treating this with simple intravenous morphine injections still persists among a small group of surgeons and anesthetists today. The concept of multimodal or a multifaceted approach to pain control is the gold standard today. Numerous studies have confirmed tremendous pain reduction and increased patient satisfaction when compared to the old techniques.

Basically, these involve a combination of three things: preventing the inflammatory "firestorm" of pain from developing, blocking pain transmission and introducing a good self-treatment regimen to control the pain after the operation.

During surgery, the release of substances from damaged tissue causes the production of pain chemicals. Like an itch that gets worse with scratching, the nerves become sensitized with repeated stimulation — to the point that any touch feels painful. In addition, changes in the spinal cord where pain signals travel can transform the pain cells there. Scientists can see changes in the DNA within the cell and changes in the release of pain chemicals.

Fortunately, drugs in pill form taken before an operation can reduce these pain chemicals. These drugs are also taken after the operation. By doing this, the "wind-up" of pain is prevented.

The next technique — blocking pain transmission — is akin to temporarily cutting the wires of a telephone grid. In this case, it means blocking pain signals along nerves with "freezing" medicines — or alternatively, blocking pain signals at the spinal cord, where they converge, by injecting drugs there (using epidural and spinal needles).

Finally, self-administration of pain medicines after the operation improves pain control. A person's satisfaction with pain control is not only dependent upon how quickly and effectively pain medicines work — it's also the psychological sense of self-control that gives people greater satisfaction. Whether it is a pain pump to self-administer pain medicines in hospital or important home instructions to quickly get on top of pain and regularly dose yourself, these all decrease your perceived pain after the operation.

Pain control is a much bigger issue than just making sure you feel comfortable. Body function is significantly affected by pain after an operation. Take, for example, two different leg operations — knee replacement surgery and anterior cruciate ligament surgery (the same operation Tiger Woods had). If there is better pain control after the operation, through the use of multimodal techniques, you will be discharged from hospital sooner, with less nausea and vomiting. You will also have superior ability to use and bend the repaired knee right after surgery.

It's important to know that better pain control has long-term benefits as well. After discharge from hospital, those who had better pain control immediately after the operation had better ability to climb stairs at home. In fact, six months and one year later, both the anterior cruciate repair and the knee replacement patients who had good pain control in the days after the operation were better able to resume normal activities. So, if you think that pain control is not an important issue, you're wrong.

Let's tackle the nausea problem. It's possible to predict your higher risk of nausea and vomiting based on five factors: if you're female, have experienced previous nausea and vomiting after surgery, are having surgery lasting longer than 30 minutes, are a nonsmoker and have a history of motion sickness. The relative chance of feeling nauseated and vomiting is 10 percent, 20 percent, 40 percent, 60 percent and 80 percent based on your having nil, one, two, three and four of these risk factors.

The chances of nausea increase more with these surgeries: plastic, eye, shoulder, gynecological (non-D&C) and dental surgeries.

Although the surgery can't be modified, much can be done to reduce nausea and vomiting through use of drugs and different anesthesic techniques. Again, like the multi-factorial plans that control pain after operations, combinations of drugs and techniques are found to be most effective.

To control nausea after discharge home, studies have advocated giving a supply of anti-nausea pills for two to three days. This significantly decreases the number of people still nauseated days after the operation.

So, the preoperative clinic and anesthesia department should explain strategies about effective pain control and prevention of nausea and vomiting, and have treatments ready for you. If they don't, you should push for answers and solutions.

One topic that hasn't had much study, and that people don't know much about, is feeling faint or passing out at home, even after minor operations. After discharge from hospital, many assume that once they're home, they will rapidly return to their normal alertness and strength. Remember, your body has been under the stress of an operation; there may be oozing from the wound and residual anesthetic effects may persist for the rest of the day. All this adds up and may make you feel queasy and weak. I've spoken to a number of patients — especially men — who seem to be predisposed to feeling faint in places like the bathroom, where they could get a bad knock to the head. Just beware, take things easy and if feeling faint, immediately try to recline and lie down to let the feeling pass. When it's time to get up, do it slowly, with some assistance.

The Last Supper

My final thoughts, before I discuss what to expect with specific operations, concern eating and drinking preoperatively. I'm surprised to find people who were told not to drink anything eight hours before surgery. Many people scheduled for afternoon surgery may experience dehydration and a severe headache because they skipped their morning coffee. Going for surgery is stressful enough without being forced to feel thirsty or suffer from caffeine withdrawal. Unfortunately, there are still uninformed doctors who give these archaic rules to patients.

For at least eight years, the societies of anesthesia across the world have adopted sensible and safe rules regarding liquids and solids for adults before surgery. Numerous studies have confirmed that the stomach is empty by the time surgery begins if these rules are followed. The American, Canadian and British anesthesiology societies have endorsed these rules: a light meal (such as toast without butter, non-fiber cereals with skim milk) can be eaten six hours prior to operation time. Clear fluid (anything you can see a newspaper through) or black tea and coffee can be drunk up to two hours prior to the operative time. Some hospitals may add an hour to the light meals and clear fluids restrictions — seven hours for light meals and three hours for clear fluids — in case the surgery is moved up by one hour.

The only exceptions to these rules are for those who are pregnant, those who are very obese and those who have had gastric banding surgery previously.

Make sure you discuss eating and drinking rules with your doctor before surgery.

Knee Replacement Surgery

There are three parts of the knee joint: the upper thighbone (femur), which bends and rubs against the lower shinbone (tibia), with the kneecap (patella) sitting on top. When the smooth, protective cartilage that covers the surface of the bones wears away, grinding and friction of the bare bone surfaces at the joint results in swelling and pain.

The surgeon makes a long cut in the front of the knee, trying to preserve most of the muscles and ligaments that tightly surround the joint. These muscles and ligaments literally hold the knee joint together and will do this for the artificial knee as well. The knee is then bent, causing the covering tissues to peel away, so that the joint pops open. The joint is normally covered with white, pearly, smooth cartilage. But, in the diseased knee, the cartilage is eroded, pitted and missing. It's easy to see why it's so painful, as bone grinds against bone.

There are five nerves that relay pain sensations from the knee joint, explaining why the knee is so sensitive to pain, and why knee replacement surgery is one of the most painful operations you can have.

The upper and lower bones of the knee are basically sculpted and resurfaced, with the aid of elaborate jigs — metallic guides that are carefully placed on the upper and lower parts of the joint. These jigs have slots through which oscillating saws — vibrating blades with serrated ends — are placed. These slotted guides enable precise cuts of the saw. This is the point of surgery that, if you close your eyes and just listen, sounds very much like a construction site, with hammering and the whining of saws and drills.

Then, the resurfaced end of the femur (thighbone) is replaced with a metallic cap, while the end of the tibia (shinbone) is replaced with a flat metal surface. A smooth, hard, plastic spacer is placed between these two metal surfaces — allowing them to contact and slide against the spacer in a friction-free way.

In most cases, epoxy cement is used to secure the metallic implants to the bone ends. It's a white, watery, glue-like substance that, when mixed and prepared, fills the O.R. with a heavy, chemical odor. Some O.R. staff members are quite bothered by the vapors, and it can trigger a headache in some workers. Less often, in younger patients with strong bones, non-cemented implants are used, anchored by screws and stuck into the central core of the bone. These latter implants must wait for the patient's bone cells to grow into them before they're fully secure.

During the operations, the surgeon will frequently comment on the softness or hardness of the bone as drilling, sawing and hammering takes place. You can hear the sound of the oscillating saw — its normally high-pitched vibrations can almost be stopped when encountering the hard, stone-like bone of younger patients. In contrast, old bone is easy to penetrate with drills and saws, and implants are easily hammered into place.

Major joint replacement surgery, like knee or hip replacement, is not for the weak and wimpy surgeon. There's a lot of physical effort involved when sawing, hammering, pulling and manipulating large limbs. It can be a real workout when it's an especially difficult, large or misshapen knee. O.R. greens are drenched in sweat when surgery's over. In fact, if weight reduction were a goal of the surgeon, a few major joint operations in a row would be good exercise.

As an aside, the only other operation that might accomplish this — and this is surprising — is liposuction. Here, the plastic surgeon must repeatedly move a suctioning metal probe to and fro and in a fanning motion under large areas of thick skin in order to vacuum fat cells out. After he completes the suctioning of a large patient, a sweating and puffing plastic surgeon colleague of mine often quips, "Paul, I don't have to go to the gym tonight. I've just done my exercise."

It's the physicality of the operation that appeals to many orthopedic surgeons. Blood is frequently splattered far and wide when metal components are pounded and hammered into place. One macho surgeon I know, half-seriously says the hammering has to make the blood "reach the O.R. lights and ceiling," before he is certain the implanted component is securely in place.

The pace of the operation slows once the metal implants are inserted. When knee implants are cemented in place, everyone must wait seven to ten minutes for the epoxy cement to harden before closure of muscle, ligaments and skin. A lump of extra cement is kept on hand and tested in order to gauge when it has hardened sufficiently. Some surgeons express their inner artistic selves by creating miniature sculptures with the cement before it hardens. I've seen some earnest attempts to depict horses, birds, flowers — as well as the occasional try at some erotic art forms.

Let's now discuss the two most common types of anesthetic for knee replacement surgery. You can either be put fully asleep under a general anesthetic, or be "frozen" from about the waist down with a spinal or epidural needle in the back, which is called regional anesthesia. I've found more people are choosing the needle in the back — a significant change from a few years ago.

There are some definite advantages to being "frozen" for knee surgery, rather than being put to sleep. During the operation, there is less stress on the heart, in terms of high blood pressure changes and fast heart rates. Some studies have indicated a small but demonstrable reduction in the likelihood of dying over the entire hospital stay, when compared to general anesthetic. After the surgery, there is a lower risk of being nauseated in the recovery room, and later on, a lower chance of getting a life-threatening blood clot in the operated leg. Subjectively, patients just look better right after surgery; they are more alert, less confused and in no immediate pain.

Whether you have a general anesthetic or regional anesthesia, pain after the surgery can be controlled when multimodal techniques, using special drugs and nerve blocks, are used.

I realize for many people, the thought of inserting a needle into the back is scary. But it really is quite safe, with a very low risk of spinal or back damage, and is not a painful procedure — pregnant women get these kinds of needles all the time for their labor pains.

After numbing drugs are injected into the back, large surgical sheets are hung as a barrier to block the patient's view of the operation. Then, the anesthetist chooses the level of sedation necessary for each patient, from the quiet, relaxed and mellow state some patients prefer to the total unawareness others need.

Having given many spinal and epidural needles, it's easy to consider it routine and become a bit blasé about the whole affair. But, if you think about it, those needles accomplish a pretty remarkable thing. The surgeon has just cut open a body part and is chiselling and sawing bone and tissue — while, on the other side of the surgical barrier, the patient is totally comfortable, moving his arms, and engaging me in a conversation about the weather. (On those occasions when bowel and gut operations are carried out, with the patient's innards spread out on the surgical field — and the only anesthesia is an epidural or spinal needle — I'm reminded of the scene from *Terminator*, where the android, though gutted and sliced in half, moves his upper arms and is still conscious.)

When having regional anesthesia, choosing the level of

sedation is important. If you don't give enough, some patients, in a marijuana-like haze, may repeatedly interrupt the surgeon, sometimes at critical moments.

"How's it going, Doc?"

"It's going just fine, Mr. Adams. Now just relax and go to sleep," the surgeon replies.

Five minutes later, "Is everything going okay, Doc?"

"Everything is fine. Just relax and try to be quiet."

Six minutes later, "Are you almost finished, Doc?"

It can be disconcerting and, frankly, irritating when a spaced-out patient tries to join the operating room team in our discussions about the latest sports scores, movies and hospital gossip.

When this happens, you can sense the level of frustration in the operating room rising. From the other side of the surgical barrier, I'm given the cut-off sign — or observe exasperated eyes rolling up to the heavens or furrowed brows expressing themselves above the surgical masks. I quickly dial up the level of sedation or face the wrath of my colleagues.

There is a continuum of depth of sedation that the anesthetist can administer to a patient. Low doses of sedation — so called "conscious sedation" — relaxes a patient, yet allows them to purposefully respond to verbal and tactile stimulation. The patient breathes on their own and blood pressure is not affected. This is the sedation level that accompanies the numbing regional anesthesia techniques during knee and hip surgeries. If the level of sedation is increased with much higher doses of drugs, then a state of general anesthesia occurs. The patient is unarousable even with painful stimulus. However, this deep level of sedation requires techniques to keep the airway from closing, and necessitates that the anesthetist push air into the lungs when spontaneous breathing stops. At this level of sedation, blood pressure frequently becomes unstable, requiring careful monitoring.

With drug overdoses, this dangerous level of general anesthesia occurs. It was likely the cause of Michael Jackson's death — a death that could possibly have been avoided with a few gentle puffs of oxygen delivered via an oxygen mask and bag.

Most people are surprised about some things concerning the recovery period after surgery. First, be aware you might be given a continuous passive motion (CPM) machine that bends and straightens your knee while in bed. Its purpose is to increase knee movement — something that can potentially be lost if scar tissue tightens and surrounds the new knee. This passive motion can be very painful for patients, unless the previously described multimodal pain options are given. It's one of the reasons that pain control is so important after knee surgery.

Also, many patients have the mistaken idea that after knee surgery, you just rest and are given a few knee exercises. Nothing could be further from the truth. In fact, numerous exercises for the knee, as well as movement of the entire body, are the two most important factors influencing recovery after knee surgery. Movement of your body prevents the development of pressure sores on the skin, leg clots and pneumonia. You'll have special exercises to do while lying in bed. On the first day after surgery, you'll be helped to a chair and while sitting, be given exercises for the knee. Assistance is given daily to walk increasingly longer distances. Again, pain control is important to allow people to move.

It's a long and hard road to recovery.

Many people say that moving with the new knee is like learning to walk all over again. Obviously, some muscles for walking have been damaged from the surgery and must heal. Also, specialized proprioceptive nerves, which help a person feel, position and orient the knee, have been cut or disrupted. The new implants confuse your body. Some patients have felt that their operated leg doesn't even belong to them. So you must get used to the feeling and orientation of the new knee in order to walk. Even swimming is different, as the implant has a different buoyancy and position in the water. In the same way, swimming with the new knee has to be relearned.

There's a lot of effort required in order to fully recover. One of the unfortunate consequences of inadequate movement is a semi-locked, scarred knee. Unless the scar tissue is broken and adequate range of motion restored, you won't be able to walk normally. The treatment for this is simple and crude: with the patient under general anesthetic, the surgeon forces the knee to bend. The disturbing sound of scar tissues being torn and ripped apart fills the operating room — like the cracking of many knuckles simultaneously. For many of us in the O.R., the sound is definitely an *ew* moment — equivalent to hearing nails scratching on a blackboard or a metal chair squeaking on the floor.

Afterwards, unless there is adequate pain control, it's an agonizing experience for the patient, as damaged nerves are reawakened and inflammatory chemicals are re-released. The whole process of rehabilitation starts all over again.

Ultimately, recovery from knee surgery is really dependent upon the effort you make to use the new knee postoperatively from the very first day.

Hip Replacement Surgery

The hip joint is composed of the round "ball" of the femur (the bone that extends from the knee to the hip) that moves within the cup-like "socket" of the pelvic bone. When the smooth cartilage coating the ball and socket is worn away, bone on bone friction causes pain. These are big bones, and so this is big surgery.

Similar to a worn-out knee, a degenerated hip joint is debilitating. It's distressing to see the suffering of patients with these worn-out joints. Even the most routine and simple tasks, such as getting up and walking across the room, are curtailed. The pain can be agonizing and, in some cases, joint degeneration progresses quickly and requires admission to the emergency room to deal with the suffering.

At the start of the surgery, the patient is first put on his or her side, with the operated hip facing up. This is not as easy as you may think. With very large patients, it can be quite a task, and urgent calls for help to turn the patient are made. At least four to five people are sometimes required in a coordinated heave-ho to safely position the patient. Bolsters are strategically and firmly placed on either side of the patient to ensure stability. There have been very unsettling cases of patients suddenly shifting during the operation or almost falling off the operating table. When situations like this occur, there is a collective gasp in the operating room, and all those around the patient quickly try to rectify the problem.

Once the surgical site has been thoroughly cleaned and disinfected, the surgeon then cuts muscles and ligaments at the side of the hip to get at the joint. Again, with very large patients, at least four or five inches of fat and tissue have to be cut before the hip is exposed. Special elongated instruments are needed in order to reach the hip joint when it lies in these cavernous recesses. Then the ball and socket of the joint are separated. As this occurs, a strange sucking sound can be heard as a vacuum that normally exists between the ball and socket is pulled apart.

In traditional hip replacement surgery, the worn-out neck and ball-end of the thighbone is cut off and removed.

Then, the hip socket is ground down and resurfaced with an ugly looking grinding instrument. It's a whining power tool with a bulbous, rotating end made up of a nasty collection of razor-like bits — it looks like it came straight out of a horror movie. Once the socket is ground down, it's replaced with an implanted socket made of plastic, metal or ceramic. Uncemented socket implants are held in place by the tightness of fit or inserted screws. Over time, bone grows into the porous structure of the implant to firmly anchor it. With cemented socket implants, the same epoxy cement used with knee replacements will anchor the socket in the pelvic bone.

Attention is now turned to the cut-off end of the thighbone. It is reamed out with long rasp-like instruments in order to create a hollow cavity in the bone. A tapered long stem resembling a blunt, curved spike made of metal is inserted into the hollowed shaft of the thighbone. If the stem is uncemented, it is held in place by its tight fit in the bone. Alternatively, epoxy cement can bond the stem to the bone.

Tremendous hammering occurs during hip surgery, when a surgeon must firmly root the artificial socket into the pelvic bone or vigorously hammer rasps into the thighbone to fit an implanted stem. Like certain points in knee surgery, but to an even greater degree, this is where blood can be sent flying across the operating room onto the masked faces of the assistants, the ceiling and lights — and most irritating to me, onto my anesthetic machine and records. After the hammering, the face masks and operating room gowns of everyone close by are covered with spots and splashes of blood — it's a very messy sight.

At this stage, because the artificial hip joint hasn't been put together, the patient's leg is loose and limp and dangles awkwardly to the side of the body like a large puppet's floppy leg, held on only by threads.

Finally, a ball made of metal or ceramic is added to the tip of the stem, and this ball is inserted into the previously implanted socket. The hip is tested for stability, then the wound is sutured and closed.

For younger patients, an option being offered at some centers is to not remove the worn-out ball-end of the thighbone, but instead resurface this ball and cover it with a metal hat. A metallic socket is inserted into the pelvic bone. If necessary, a standard hip replacement can be done later.

This technique of resurfacing the hip bone, instead of replacing it, gives younger patients better range of motion of the hip joint and so allows them to participate in more vigorous activities. However, the operative technique is more difficult, and there may be a higher breakdown rate of the hip joint after a few years. Thus, for older patients — who don't need the extra range of motion for routine daily activities, and for whom a second operation (if the resurfacing technique fails) is more stressful — a standard hip operation is better.

As far as anesthesia for hip replacement is concerned, there is definite evidence demonstrating the superiority of a regional anesthetic, with a spinal or epidural needle in the back, over a general anesthetic. There is less blood loss and a decreased need for a blood transfusion, a lower chance of developing a clot in the leg and less pain.

Again, when having regional anesthesia, an appropriate level of sedation is given, so that you don't have to be aware of the hammering, drilling and sawing that occurs during the operation.

The recovery period after hip replacement emphasizes getting moving and trying to walk on the first day after surgery. At least twice daily, you'll be assisted to get out of bed to walk a bit and transfer to a chair. In the same way as after knee surgery, early movement avoids pressure sores, leg clots and pneumonia.

Overall, pain after hip replacement is not as severe as the pain after knee replacement operations.

Because some muscles have been cut and pulled during the hip surgery, specific exercises are given to strengthen damaged muscles. The stress of large operations like hip replacement causes the body to become deconditioned. Muscle mass throughout the body, not just at the hips, decreases and you become less fit postoperatively. Biochemical markers in the blood show that your body actually catabolizes — that is, breaks down — muscle tissue in response to an operation. Many people complain that they feel so tired and weak after this operation and catabolism is one of the main reasons for this.

That's why it's so important to get up and move after surgery, in order to regain fitness and muscle mass as well as get used to the new hip implant.

Cystoscopic Surgery

Some people experience flank pain or pain when urinating. Others have trouble with a slow urine stream or feel they never completely empty their bladders. Blood could be detected in the urine. All these conditions may require an examination of the urinary plumbing. This is what a cystoscopic examination does. Urine is made in the kidneys, flows through the straw-like ureters, then empties into the balloon-shaped, urine-collecting bladder. In men, urine empties from the bladder, passing by the prostate gland and then out through the urethra and penis. In women, the organs are the same, obviously minus the prostate and penis. Cystoscopic procedures can examine and treat these parts of the urinary system.

During cystoscopic surgery, the legs are placed in stirrups. Most women have had their legs in stirrups before. For most men, it's a new experience.

Men are also a little more squeamish about cystoscopic procedures than women, since it involves introducing a scope into their penis. During the procedure, they'll probably be surrounded by at least two to three lovely urological nurses, who assist during the procedure. Exposing themselves to these lovely women, with feet up in stirrups, waiting to have an object pushed into the penis, has been described by some men as a "psychologically challenging" experience.

But as they say, once you come into hospital, male or female, you've got to leave all modesty at the door.

The urologist can use two different types of scopes. Both types are inserted into the penis or urethra to look into the urinary system. The first is a flexible scope about the thickness of a pencil with a fiber-optic scope and light. Usually, no general anesthetic is required, because freezing gel, squeezed into the penis or urethra, is adequate. However, after the procedure, there can be an uncomfortable burning sensation upon urination that can last for a few days. It's caused by the irritation of the scope.

The second type of scope, the rigid scope, is a different beast. Having a diameter ranging from a quarter-of-an-inch to almost half-an-inch (.56 cm to .9 cm), inserted through the penis or urethra, can be very uncomfortable for many patients, even with lubricating and numbing gel. Many would advise a general anesthetic or, if appropriate, a spinal or regional anesthetic when the rigid scope is used. Before the use of the smaller flexible scopes, it was not uncommon to hear a lot of yelping and screaming when rigid scopes were inserted without general anesthetics.

Whereas flexible scopes are adequate for examining your urinary system, rigid scopes have side ports through which various instruments can be inserted, giving urologists more options to treat various conditions. Abnormal tissue in the prostate and bladder can be cauterized with electric currents or can be lasered. Small grabbers can be directed by rigid scopes into the bladder or ureter to snag stones. Stents can be introduced through the ureters into the kidneys.

Most cystoscopy cases are very safe and routine. But there are notable deviations from the routine where interesting side effects involving penises and bladders occur.

The first concerns the effects cystoscopy can have on young men. Even under general anesthetic, the introduction of scopes through the penises of young men can be very stimulating. Their bodies are full of raging hormones, and the nerves around the penises are at their most sensitive. Though the patient is asleep, Mr. Penis is awake and ready for action. Even the introduction of numbing gel or the application of sterilizing solution on or near the penis can produce a very full erection during, for example, hernia surgeries and appendectomies.

In the O.R. we confess to a cruel rite of indoctrination, inflicted upon the innocent rookie nurses, making use of this well-known physiologic reaction. During their first days in the operating room, we ask them to sterilize these surgical areas.

"Oh, by the way, Anna, why don't you apply some iodine to the surgical area? We want to assess your sterilization techniques."

We stand back and mischievously observe their stunned reaction when the penis comes alive — throbbing, rising and pointing.

"My, my, what have you done, Anna? ... You've got a very special technique ... Nice touch. ... Anna, you really know how to please the patients."

For the urologist looking down through the inserted scope, other than the awkwardness of the situation — a large erection pointing at his face — there are practical issues to deal with. The rigid cystoscope is approximately 9 inches in length (23 centimeters). The cystoscope must be long enough to be inserted through the length of the penis plus traverse the prostate in order to get a view of the inside of the bladder. For the average sized male, you can see that this would not pose a serious problem. However, for the very well endowed . . .

I can recall a case I did with a urologist some years ago. We had just begun a rigid cystoscopy on a young man. Suddenly, I heard the urologist say, "Paul, can you do something about this?"

I looked up to see him struggling with a very, very large, erect penis, trying desperately to push the cystoscope deeper though the scope seemed buried to its hilt.

Over the next 30 minutes, we tried every pharmacological and physiological method to make the beast go flaccid, without success. It was like a large, stubborn snake displaying itself with throbbing pride after having just devoured the scope. Finally, we decided to take the scope out and let time do its work. Without the stimulation of the scope, after some minutes, it gave up its preening stand and we were able to proceed. For the rest of the day, our case was the talk of the O.R.

On another occasion, a urologist was struggling with another erection, trying to manipulate the scope deeper. It seemed as though he was almost fighting with the penis — cursing, weaving the scope to and fro, in and out or side to side. We could see he wanted to wrestle this penis into flaccid submission. Suddenly he shouted, "What's this stuff?" A white substance spewed out of the penis. He paused, and then, red faced, the answer came to him. "It's semen. I guess I moved the scope a little too much."

At that moment, most of us in the room didn't need to hear this, having witnessed the vigorous penile manipulations — "Gee, Mr. Urologist, you really think so?" Regardless, this episode could aptly be described as an inadvertent floggin' the log and examination session.

Another interesting side effect occurs when bladder tumors are cauterized on the lateral (side) walls of the bladder. Because the obturator nerve runs just outside the lateral walls of the bladder, it can accidentally be stimulated when the electric cautery is applied on the bladder wall. It's the obturator nerve connected to the inner thigh muscles that allows you to squeeze your legs together.

During cystoscopic operations, the urologist's head is situated between the stirruped legs of the patient, allowing him to peer through the scope. You can see the urologist is in a particularly dangerous spot if one leg were to suddenly jump off the stirrups towards the midline.

While watching the urologist work cauterizing bladder tissue, you sometimes see the legs twitching dangerously inwards with each burn. It reminds me of a person with his head between the jaws of a deadly trap that's ready to spring and snap closed. I hold my breath with each burn and think to myself — "Man, urology can sometimes be a risky specialty."

In fact, about ten percent of lateral bladder tumor cauterizations will stimulate this nerve. It can be very strange to see a fully asleep patient knock the urologist on the head with powerful jerks of the leg. To stop this, the urologist will ask me to give muscle relaxants to fully paralyze the patient. If I don't give enough, I get dirty looks.

Though the majority of cystoscopic cases proceed unremarkably, there are some unusual events that occur, helping to break up the monotony of the day.

Hernia Surgery

Hernias are basically weaknesses in the wall of the abdomen that bulge and cause pain. There is the potential for sections of the gut to be pushed out and trapped in these weaknesses. There are three basic ways for hernias to be surgically repaired. Two methods fix the problem from outside the body, and the third fixes it from the inside.

The first is the traditional method of sewing abdominal wall layers together to close the defect. This is the type of procedure done at many hospitals.

The second way is to sew a patch of plastic over the defect.

The final repair method is to do it from the inside of the abdominal wall. After inflating the abdominal cavity with gas, keyhole incisions allow the introduction of grapplers, which manipulate a plastic mesh to cover the hernia defects on the inner abdominal wall. This mesh is stapled onto the wall. This method has been shown to have the least postoperative pain, compared to the external repairs.

Surgeons can be quite vocal in arguing the advantages and disadvantages of each technique. However, in most cases, the quality of the repair is more dependent upon the experience and skill of the surgeon than on the technique itself.

With the first two external surgical techniques, the surgeon can make the repairs without having to put the patient to sleep.

If the hernia is not too large, the simplest approach is to inject freezing around the area of the surgery. The patient avoids getting all the drugs of a general anesthetic, has a smaller chance of being nauseated, gets good pain control after the operation and avoids the grogginess of a general anesthetic. Overall, it is the safest approach.

The downside for the surgeon is that he or she must work slowly, freezing the operative areas incrementally while cutting and suturing.

The patient may feel twinges of the needle and some minor discomfort with pulling and tugging of deeper tissues. It's not severe pain and extra freezing can always be added.

A second way external repairs can be done by regional anesthesia is to insert needles in the back and inject medicines that freeze the body from the waist down.

Finally, with internal hernia repairs, where gas is used to inflate the abdominal cavity, the patient must be put to sleep.

An interesting side effect occurs in men, when the gas in the abdominal cavity travels through tissue planes, down to the scrotum and penis. The gas inflates this area like a balloon, so by the end of surgery, the penis and scrotum expand to three or four times normal size. This resolves in about 30 minutes, with no ill effects. In the meantime, when someone in the O.R. who has never seen this asks how the patient will feel about this, our usual answer is "very proud."

The Caesarean Section

I'll describe what occurs when a woman has a Caesarean section under regional anesthetic. This involves the insertion of a spinal or epidural needle into the back, with the injection of medicines that numb the nerves that exit the spinal cord. The anesthetist tries to achieve numbness from below the nipple in order for the patient to be comfortable throughout the procedure. The risks of needle insertion in the back are very low. Chances of permanently damaging the spinal cord and nerves that exit from the spinal cord have been calculated to be less than one in 80,000 to 100,000.

This is the most common way that Caesarean sections are anesthetized in North America. It has been shown to be the safest for mother and child. Additionally, because other long-lasting analgesic medicines can also be injected, there is better pain control with regional anesthetics compared to general anesthetics.

The only negatives associated with regional anesthesia are more frequent shivering and nausea as compared to the general anesthetic.

There are higher risks of complications when giving a general anesthetic to a pregnant patient. Basically, these risks are associated with delivering and maintaining oxygen to the mother. Because pregnancy causes a change to the tongue and throat, placing breathing tubes into the lungs for general anesthetics is more difficult. Also, because the mother is breathing for both herself and the baby, oxygen is rapidly used up from her lungs. It is frightening to see how fast a pregnant woman's lips will change from bright pink to dark blue when there is any difficulty delivering oxygen to the lungs.

Thin women, with easily identifiable bony prominences in their back, make insertion of the epidural and spinal needles easy. However, with increasing weight, it becomes more challenging. Sometimes with very heavy women, it's more a "best guess" method to locate the proper point to insert the needle.

It's completely natural to be very nervous before a Caesarean section. To be totally relaxed would be abnormal. However, terrified patients present the greatest challenge. Cleansing of the back, or injection of a small amount of local anesthetic, can cause some people to jump and jerk away. Unfortunately, when precise placement of a needle near the spinal cord is important, it makes the procedure especially dangerous. The best advice is to be as calm and still as possible. The insertion of the needle is not a painful procedure.

Once the epidural drugs have been injected, the woman is asked to lie down. Anesthetic monitors are applied. Surgical draw sheets are erected so the woman doesn't have to watch the operation. The surgeon will carefully pinch and probe at the incision site to ensure everything is frozen. The surgery can then begin.

Although patients are frozen and won't feel pain beneath the nipple-line, many still feel touching and pulling sensations during surgery. Don't panic. These sensations will only occur a few times during surgery.

There are three side effects that frequently occur during a Caesarean section under regional anesthetic. The first is shivering. Occasionally, the shivering can be so severe that it almost resembles a seizure. Women shiver because they are cold and frightened and because the medication injected near the spine triggers this response. Most anesthetists will give patients warmed fluids and blankets to help maintain body temperature.

The second side effect is a sensation of being short of breath. Because the spinal or epidural prevents patients from feeling their chest expand as they breathe, some feel like they're suffocating.

Here is an important tip for women. If you can talk normally, then you're breathing normally. It also sometimes helps to blow into the oxygen mask, in order to feel the breath against your face. This should reassure you that your breathing is normal.

The final side effect is nausea and vomiting. In most cases this occurs because the blood pressure has fallen after the spinal or epidural medicines are injected. A slight fall in blood pressure is a normal occurrence. However, larger reductions in blood pressure cause pregnant women to feel nauseated. A vigilant anesthetist will watch the blood pressure carefully and give medicines to temporarily elevate low blood pressures in order to prevent nausea. A helpful thing women can do is to immediately inform the anesthetist of any nausea symptoms. In that way, blood pressure–elevating medicines can be given right away.

A combination of all three side effects can certainly panic some women. Unfortunately, sedative drugs cannot be given during a Caesarean section because they easily enter the baby's blood. The baby will then have breathing problems.

During the operation, I try to reassure women as much as possible and tell them to enjoy their newborn child. As any parent knows, the brief side effects experienced during the operation pale in comparison to the challenges of helping baby to grow up.

CHAPTER 7

Everything You Ever Wanted to Know About Anesthesia
(But Were Too Unconscious to Ask)

In this section, I've collected and answered questions that many patients have asked me about anesthesia, surgery and the operating room. I hope these will answer many questions you may have as well.

I'm really nervous about my surgery. Isn't there anything that they can give me to relax while I wait?

In the past, sedation was routinely given about an hour or two prior to surgery. An intramuscular injection of morphine or Demerol, along with Gravol or some other anti-nausea drug, was given. Ativan or some other tranquilizer was an option.

Today, sedation is not routinely given because it might prolong recovery time and delay your discharge. Also, from a medical–legal standpoint, your medical history and consent must be obtained while you're not under the influence of drugs.

However, if you feel that you really need sedation, it should be discussed the day before surgery. Then they can give a preoperative order for a sublingual (under the tongue) Ativan tablet or a similar sedative. If more powerful sedation is needed, intramuscular injection of drugs like morphine and Demerol can be ordered preoperatively.

I drink five to seven strong cups of coffee a day. I get terrible headaches if I don't drink my morning coffee, and I get low blood sugar in the afternoon if I don't eat. My surgery is booked in the late afternoon. I've been told not to eat anything after midnight the day before surgery. What can I do to not feel miserable before surgery?

In the chapter "On the Table," I discussed preoperative fasting guidelines of the American, Canadian and British Anesthesia Societies.

For non-pregnant adults (without previous gastric banding surgery or severe acid reflux) a light meal, consisting of non-fiber cereals and skim milk, can be eaten six hours prior to the booked surgical time. Clear, thin fluids (like apple juice, cranberry juice, water, pop, tea and coffee without milk) can be drunk up until two hours prior to the actual surgery time. These rules should help you avoid headache and low sugar. Note: individual hospitals may increase times to seven hours for a light meal and three hours for clear fluids prior to the surgical time. This is a safety buffer, in case surgery is moved ahead by an hour.

Many surgeons and anesthetists are still living in the dark ages, inflicting needless suffering by not allowing drinking and eating after midnight the day prior to surgery. Make sure you discuss this matter with a surgeon and anesthetist before your surgery.

Hopefully your surgeon and anesthetist are up to date, so that you can enjoy your cups of java in the morning, along with some early morning cereal.

I'm really scared of needles. They really hurt a lot. I know that my nephew, who was five years old when he had his surgery, was "gassed" to sleep with the anesthetic machine instead of having an intravenous started. Why can't I get the gas?

There are many people who panic when thinking about an intravenous needle. Some have been jabbed many times because they have small, inaccessible veins. They come into the operating room terrified it's going to be difficult again, and unfortunately it usually is. Their fear, lack of fluids and the cold temperatures in the operating room make the veins collapse more.

As I mentioned earlier, a second group consists of men with tattoos all over their body who are also frequently anxious. You'd think they'd be used to needles, but many of them are petrified of them.

Pre-teenage girls of 11 or 12 years old are pillars of strength when an intravenous is started. Boys at this age are the opposite; they're uncooperative and terrified. The challenge is to keep them still enough to insert the intravenous.

Some adults think it's possible for them to go under anesthetic gases to avoid the needle poke. However, as a person breathes the gas, they may become confused and thrash around or become violent. While a five-year-old can be held and controlled, large adults can be dangerous. I've seen nurses and doctors get punched. It can be scary. So, unless you weigh 60 pounds or less, you're going to get a needle.

There are ways sympathetic anesthetists can make the process less painful. They can find the smallest gauge needle to poke you with. Contrary to what many men think, size does matter. Also, they can insert the needle in less sensitive places, like in the bend of the elbow, as opposed to back of the hand. Even pre-insertion techniques, such as stretching the skin or having the person cough and rapidly poking the skin, as opposed to using a slow, deliberate push, will make for a less painful experience.

So what can you do to make things better for yourself? If you've had difficult veins in the past, inform the anesthetist. They can give you nitrous oxide (laughing gas) while they insert the needle, to create a less painful and more relaxed experience for you and the anesthetist. They can place warm blankets over the arm, which will cause the veins to expand. Also, if one arm has had more success (many times, one arm is better for an intravenous) or if a certain vein has been used successfully in the past (some people call this their money vein), show the anesthetist. Finally, at the drugstore, you can purchase a numbing cream called EMLA. It will completely numb the skin if applied at least two hours before the poke. (Note: please apply to areas where there are good veins. We've had people apply cream two hours before to areas with no veins. EMLA is not useful under those circumstances.)

Using all the methods described above, there's hope that your intravenous insertion will be painless and accomplished on the first try.

I've got some dental work on the tips of my front teeth. I've also got a tooth implant. Do I have to worry that these could be damaged during my anesthetic?

Damage to teeth is the most common malpractice claim against anesthetists, so we're a little sensitive about this issue. Once you fall asleep with a general anesthetic, the most important job of the anesthetist is to make sure that oxygen can be delivered to the lungs. In order to do this, devices are inserted into the mouth through which oxygen is delivered. When these devices are inserted, they can cause damage to the teeth.

There are generally two types of devices used today. The first is called a laryngeal mask. Think of a soft, rubbery, half-pear-shaped object inserted into the back of the throat, attached to a hollow tube that exits the mouth. This hollow tube is connected to the anesthesia machine, to deliver oxygen and gases into the patient. The invention of this device has made anesthesiology much safer, not only because it's easy to insert this soft object into the back of the throat, but because there's minimal risk to the teeth.

The older, traditional way to deliver gases and oxygen to the patient was to place a breathing tube directly into the windpipe using an L-shaped metal device inserted into the mouth.

This L-shaped device rests near the teeth. So having a small receding chin and expensive front dental work puts the teeth at risk. If there's a small-jawed Peewee Herman–type patient with new dental implants coming for surgery, you'll have an anxious anesthetist.

I'm going for major shoulder surgery. I'd like to know if I'm going to feel a lot of pain when I wake up. Is there anything that can be done to prevent this pain?

There have been lots of studies rating the expected pain after various operations. It's always a good thing to know, so your surgeon and anesthetist can work together to maximally decrease discomfort. You should never resign yourself to suffering after operations. With good planning, much can be done not only to decrease the pain you might feel immediately upon awakening, but also to decrease the cumulative total pain in the days after the operation.

You should expect minor pain after minor urological and gynecological operations and skin operations (other than burn debridement).

You should expect moderate pain after ear and nose operations, thyroidectomy, inguinal hernia and appendectomy, hip operations and laparoscopic gallbladder surgery.

You should expect major pain after shoulder operations, knee replacement, open kidney operations and open bowel operations. (Open means a large cut through the body wall, not keyhole surgery.)

After your shoulder surgery, expect pretty bad pain upon

awakening and for the next 24 hours afterwards. Pain is the worst in the first 24 hours after surgery, then decreases afterwards.

Fortunately, now that you know this, a plan to significantly decrease this pain can be developed with the cooperation of your doctors (if there are no medical contraindications or possible side effects). A few hours before the surgery, you could take a combination of drugs like naproxen and acetaminophen (to decrease the release of pain-activating chemicals from the body) and gabapentin (to decrease your sensitivity to pain).

You could also have a nerve block to numb the shoulder before the surgery starts. With a successful nerve block, you wouldn't have pain for hours after surgery. But, in anticipation of later pain, you would have a supply of prescribed narcotics to take on a regular basis at the first signs of pain. Don't wait until it's unbearable or you'll always be playing catch-up, and remember to take them regularly. Bowel softeners and lots of fiber in the diet are really important to prevent constipation. In addition, you'll be prescribed gabapentin, acetaminophen and naproxen, the same drugs you took before surgery, to take for the next two days.

By doing all these things, not only will you have less pain, but the rehabilitation of your shoulder and your return to normal activities will be much faster.

I weigh over 300 pounds and have sleep apnea. I'm scheduled for minor surgery. Are there any concerns?

I don't mean to frighten you, but you're one of those patients who really scare doctors and nurses in the operating room.

I know that being very overweight is difficult for you in daily life, but it also creates a whole series of problems in the O.R.

First, there are practical considerations, like making sure the extra-large operating table is ready and the large stretcher for transport is available after the operation.

Blood-pressure cuffs may not work accurately, or at all, on very large arms. Even starting an intravenous can be a struggle because veins are frequently buried under the skin.

Just after the sleep drugs are injected, there is a very small time window to insert a breathing tube into your windpipe because obese people use up oxygen faster and have less oxygen in their lungs. After they're put asleep, their faces can change from a well-oxygenated pink, to a pre–cardiac arrest blue in a matter of minutes. Unfortunately, inserting breathing tubes in obese people is technically harder.

After the breathing tube is inserted, the ventilators on the anesthesia machine will struggle to push oxygen into lungs that are compressed by a large belly.

While sleeping, obese people have a higher risk of developing nerve injuries due to pressure on nerves in the arms because of the weight of the arms. Extra padding to nerves, especially at the elbows, is important.

Performing a regional anesthetic with a needle in the back is often impossible. Extra-long needles, six to eight inches in length, are not easily inserted into the back due to thick layers of fat and tissue.

The surgeon has to cut through thick layers of skin and fat using long instruments and large retractors to keep these layers away from the operative site. It's just technically more challenging to work in a deep hole where the surgeon has to struggle to get things done. There's usually a lot of cursing behind the surgeon's mask.

After surgery is complete, it takes a team of four to five people to safely transfer the patient from the operating table onto the stretcher. Obese patients are at a higher risk of falling off the operating table.

In the recovery room, oxygen levels are more difficult to maintain due to the fact that the patient's large abdomen squeezes into his or her lungs. Recovery is slower because it's hard to move around. For obese patients, there's increased risk of forming blood clots in the legs and a higher postoperative infection rate.

Finally, it can be hazardous for doctors to operate on large patients. A very obese woman came for minor vaginal surgery. Because of her weight and other health issues, we decided a general anesthetic was dangerous and that light sedation would be safer. We started an intravenous with great difficulty and injected her with sedative drugs. She was breathing peacefully and unaware with a contented smile upon her face. Her legs were placed in lithotomy position — feet suspended and legs spread apart. The gynecologist sat between the legs and began an examination. Suddenly, the woman's massive thighs clamped down hard, tightly trapping the head of the hapless doctor. The sight of the poor man — head totally enveloped between two huge thighs, arms waving frantically at his side, emitting muffled cries of "Help, help!" — was overwhelming for the rest of us.

So, if you are truly obese — which is the case if your weight in kilograms divided by your height in meters squared is greater than 30 — and if there is enough time, you should really consider losing as much weight as possible prior to surgery under the supervision of your G.P. I guarantee that with each pound you lose, the risk of complications will decrease, as will the anxiety of everybody in the operating room.

I'm a family doctor and I'm booked for an operation. It's going to be hard for me to not question and suggest things be done a certain way, given that I am a physician. How can I inform everyone in the operating room, recovery room and the ward that I want things done my way?

Look buddy, just because you're a doctor doesn't mean you know how things work in the operating room. Physicians can be the most irritating patients to look after. A little knowledge can easily be mistaken for expertise. Even physician specialists working outside their area of practice are ignorant about what goes on in other specialties.

I remember a real pain-in-the-neck physician who was booked for a major operation. He insisted on questioning and sometimes opposing every preoperative order. He frequently shooed the pre-op nurse away. After the operation, he was constantly pressing his bedside nurse call button for inappropriate reasons. I know how important it is for patients to speak up and be heard in order to get better care, but in this case his attempts were just irritating. Only after the operating surgeon read him the riot act — by threatening to complain to the college of physicians and surgeons — did he quiet down and cooperate.

Will I dream while asleep under general anesthetic?

A recent article in the journal *Anesthesiology* showed that almost one out of five people can recall a dream after a general anesthetic. This was not related to awareness or light anesthesia. A brain wave monitor measuring the brain's electrical activity ensured that a consistent depth of anesthesia was maintained. The dreams were pleasant and focused on familiar people and experiences, such as family, friends and work. Young men with a history of remembering their dreams at home are most likely to recall dreams after surgery.

In about 2 to 3 percent of general anesthetics, a patient will dream about having surgery and will confuse this for awareness during the surgery. In most cases, the patients eventually realize it really was just a dream. There were no serious psychological consequences. True awareness under anesthetic occurs in less than one-tenth of a percent of cases. Further details about this subject are available in the chapter "A Day in the Operating Room."

While I'm asleep, what does the anesthetist actually do? Does he or she just make sure I'm asleep and my blood pressure is fine during the operation? Does the anesthetist constantly have eyes glued to the anesthetic monitor, or does he or she occasionally read the newspaper or fill out a puzzle?

Many anesthetists have compared giving an anesthetic to flying a plane. Just as takeoff is a critical moment for a pilot, so too is putting a patient to sleep — called induction — for an anesthetist. Making sure a plane's takeoff is smooth parallels making sure the blood pressure, pulse and oxygen level are stable as a patient goes to sleep. The risks of something going wrong as you fall asleep are summarized as follows:

Blood pressure: If the blood pressure falls too low, which can happen with the injection of sleep medicine, the body may go into shock with low blood flow to the brain and heart, causing damage. If the blood pressure becomes too high, which happens when breathing tubes are inserted into the airway, a patient could have a stroke or heart attack.

Heart rate: The heart rate can change tremendously as you go to sleep. Slow heart rates can send the body into shock. Fast heart rates can cause a heart attack.

Oxygen levels: Once you fall deeply asleep, breathing stops, so a device must be inserted into the airway to deliver oxygen to the lungs. The anesthetist has only a few minutes to do this once you stop breathing before the oxygen levels become critical.

Once the plane is off the ground and cruising, the pilot uses electronic displays to monitor the flight. Similarly, the anesthesia machine continuously displays all the vital signs. The anesthetic machine also constantly delivers oxygen and sleep gases to the patient. During this part of the surgery, anesthetists make sure you're kept warm, that any blood loss is replaced and that your kidneys, heart and brain are protected.

Blood pressure, heart rhythm, oxygen levels, exhaled gases, temperature, brain activity and muscle paralysis are constantly monitored on the anesthetic display as follows:

+ The blood pressure is automatically measured and displayed on the screen every two to five minutes. A pressure monitor is like an artificial finger wrapped around the arm feeling for a pulse, which indicates blood pressure.

+ The beating heart constantly produces small electrical signals seen on the monitor and measured with skin electrodes placed on the chest. The changes in shape of the electrical signal indicate an abnormal rhythm or a heart attack.

+ Oxygen levels are constantly monitored with a probe shining light on the skin to assess color (actually, it's the color of the blood flowing through the skin). This probe measures the amount of red to show if you're getting enough oxygen.

+ The oxygen level in the skin is recorded as a number and each pulse is given a musical note; a higher musical pitch means higher oxygen levels.

+ Skin electrodes placed on the forehead measure brain electrical activity and display a number from zero to 100. Alarms ring for numbers above 60, indicating possible awareness during the operation.

+ A device placed on your wrist measures how much your fingers move when stimulated with a small electric current, showing how paralyzed you are during the operation.

+ Measurements of a patient's breaths confirm that all the breathing circuits are intact. If no exhaled breaths are detected, an alarm sounds to warn of a possible disconnect.

All these vital signs are shown on a brightly lit screen, made up of colored moving lines, waves and important numbers. Alarms are set to go off if any of the vital signs are abnormal.

If a plane is stable during a flight, does the pilot constantly stare at his monitors during a very long trip? No. He sometimes will look at manuals during the flight, talk to the copilot about his favorite sports team or perhaps he will even read an article that may not be entirely related to air flight. The pilot on a long flight is comparable to anesthetists during long surgical procedures. We are constantly aware of the monitor, glancing at it every few minutes, and attuned to the beeps and possible alarms in the background — present and available to take care of problems at a moment's notice — but we're definitely not staring at the screen the entire time. Anyone would go nuts doing this during an entire case.

For very unstable, sick patients, or for complex operations, the anesthetist is constantly occupied. It's similar to a flight through major turbulence. We only have time to briefly check the monitors because we're too busy keeping things from crashing.

Now it's time to land the plane. A pilot carefully controls altitude and speed when landing and makes sure landing gear is ready to touch the ground. The anesthetist carefully controls blood pressure and pulse as the patient wakes, and makes sure the patient is able to breathe on his or her own. In addition, a smooth landing for an anesthetist means a patient wakes up without pain or nausea, which is accomplished by injecting freezing medicines and giving anti-nausea drugs.

So, to finally answer your questions, the anesthetist has a lot to do when a patient falls asleep and wakes up, and a lot to watch and monitor during surgery. The anesthetist may not look at the monitor the whole time, but he or she is constantly aware of the patient's vital signs.

I know that women can have Caesarean sections with an epidural needle in the back to freeze their lower body without having to go to sleep. Are there many other operations that can be done this way?

Excluding liver and heart transplants and lung or major intestinal surgery, almost every kind of operation can be performed without a general anesthetic. This is done by inserting needles around the spine or by injecting local anesthetics around specific nerves.

After inserting an epidural needle at the base of the neck,

then injecting numbing medicines, the sternum (chest bone) can be cut open with a saw for heart valve replacement or coronary bypass surgery. Throughout the surgery, the patient is only sedated. This same technique allows any kind of breast surgery to be done without a general anesthetic. The surgeon can remove thyroid glands, clear blockages to carotid vessels (to prevent strokes) and perform other neck operations by using local anesthetics rather than a general anesthetic.

A patient can be operated on awake for many brain operations after freezing the scalp, because brain tissue carries no pain receptors. Of course, feet, knees, hips and prostates can be frozen after injecting local anesthetics into spinal or epidural needles. We can freeze the shoulder, arm and hand with needles injected into the neck or upper arm. In fact, many shoulder operations in the United States are done this way, with the patient sedated.

The decision to perform surgery with sedation and freezing techniques depends on three factors: first, the anatomy and medical conditions allow needles to be safely inserted; second, the surgeon and anesthetist have the proper experience; finally, the patient has the confidence to undergo this technique.

This last point is important. I recall a patient who demanded to be awake for a minor knee operation. After the knee was fully numbed, the surgery began. Within minutes, even after mild sedation, he suddenly had second thoughts and started to panic. Terror filled his eyes, sweat formed on his face and his pulse and blood pressure soared. He started thrashing his arms and legs wildly. We needed to quickly convert to full general anesthetic. It could have become a very dangerous situation. It illustrates that a confident and well-informed patient is essential.

I'm having a gallbladder operation. Blood transfusions worry me. I just don't like the idea of someone else's blood in me. What are the chances that I'll need a blood transfusion?

The chance you're going to need a blood transfusion is very low for this type of surgery. Unless a large blood vessel is accidentally cut, the amount of blood loss during gallbladder surgery is minimal.

Of course, bigger operations involving many blood vessels or large areas oozing blood have a higher chance of requiring a transfusion. For example, knee surgery has about a 16 percent chance and hip replacement has a 13 percent chance of requiring a transfusion after surgery.

The chances of needing a transfusion depend on the initial hemoglobin level (red blood concentration level). Obviously, the higher the hemoglobin level, the greater the amount of blood a patient can lose before reaching a critical point.

A hemoglobin concentration of 8 grams per liter is the point where transfusion of blood should be considered in most people. Below this concentration of red blood cells, oxygen is not optimally transported throughout the body. Normal hemoglobin levels are approximately 14 to 15 grams per liter. Thus, you must lose almost 40 percent of your blood volume before transfusion is needed.

The chance of being infected by AIDS or hepatitis is very low with modern screening techniques. For example, the chance that a unit of blood contains HIV is approximately one in two million.

That being said, the decision to give a patient blood when they're on the operating table is not taken lightly. It's been shown that each unit of blood transfused increases the chance of developing a postoperative infection. It's believed that blood transfusions cause a permanent dampening of the immune system. This was first observed when kidney transplants began. Patients who received transfusions during their transplant operation had a decreased chance of rejecting the new kidney, because parts of the immune system were suppressed.

Another concern is that each unit of blood transfused during a cancer surgery may increase the chance of cancer returning. Again, modification of the immune system may be at fault.

This does not mean all transfusions are bad. A transfusion can be a life-saving treatment. However, whenever a transfusion can be avoided, most physicians will err on the side of caution. Doctors are comfortable to permit hemoglobin levels to fall to levels just above the critical point in a healthy patient, knowing the human body's recuperative powers.

One way to avoid the risks of blood transfusion before bigger operations is to *auto donate* your blood — that is, about a month before surgery, come in twice to donate your own blood and have it stored. Your body will usually replace this blood by the date of your surgery. This way, if blood is needed during surgery, you can be given your own. If you're considering this, you must plan, with the assistance of the surgeon and hospital, well in advance of the operation.

An easier way to reduce the chance of transfusion is to

build up your red blood cells weeks before the operation. Iron supplements and other drugs can increase the starting hemoglobin levels so that you can lose more blood during surgery before needing a transfusion.

Blood loss can be reduced during surgery as well. A surgeon can operate meticulously, carefully sewing vessels and cauterizing oozing tissues. The anesthetist can lower a patient's blood pressure and reduce the blood flow to cut tissue.

After my surgery, do I have to go to the recovery room? If so, what happens there and how long do I have to stay?

If you're given any sedation or have a general anesthetic, you'll go to the recovery room after surgery. When you first enter the recovery room, your vital signs — blood pressure, pulse, breathing, oxygen level and level of consciousness — are closely monitored. In the first 30 minutes after surgery, these vital signs can change rapidly. Trained nurses are alert for any instability. Occasionally, as a patient emerges from anesthetic, pain and anxiety causes his or her blood pressure to rise and heart rates to speed up. A combination of sedatives and drugs will be used to control the pain and blood pressure.

The two most common concerns are pain and nausea. The multimodal approaches to pain and nausea, discussed previously, will minimize these issues. Remember to speak up if you are suffering. The sooner your problems are dealt with, the more effective the treatment. There is no reward for being stoic. The recovery room nurses are there to help you. Nothing would make them happier than a stable, pain-free and happy patient.

When some people awaken from a general anesthetic they have an atypical reaction. Young children, teenagers and a small percentage of adults can wake up in an agitated state. Some come to shouting and punching, yet later have no recollection of doing this. If you have done this in the past, you should mention it during the preoperative assessment, so staff are aware and they can have sedatives ready.

Discharge from the recovery room is based on the Aldrete score system. Respiration, circulation, consciousness, activity and oxygen levels are given numbers from zero to two, with a total score of nine or greater indicating the patient can be safely discharged. Most recovery rooms have a 30-minute minimum stay policy. If you've had minor surgery, like removal of a skin lesion with freezing and sedation, you may be discharged in just over 30 minutes. With larger surgeries, it's common to stay in the recovery room for at least one to two hours.

When I'm on the hospital ward after my operation, should I have someone other than the ward nurse looking in on me as I recover?

It's essential to have a friend or relative speak on your behalf as you recover on the ward. The experiences of a surgeon who underwent major abdominal surgery for pancreatic cancer demonstrate why it's important. The surgery was done at a large downtown hospital where, years before, he had trained as a resident, and it went well.

After spending some time in the intensive care unit, he was transferred to the recovery ward. Unfortunately, on the day of transfer, his wife and son could only visit once in the morning and later in the evening.

He had a bladder catheter — a tube inserted into the bladder used to measure and empty urine. There was discomfort in his lower abdomen since his transfer. He could feel his bladder becoming increasingly full. It was obvious the catheter was blocked, causing the urine to accumulate. He called and complained to the ward nurse. However, when she investigated, she just looked at the catheter and muttered, "I see urine; it's still draining." As his pain increased, he repeatedly called the nursing station. His complaints were ignored.

He was eventually in severe agony, and called his friend, the chief of urology at another hospital, to help him. When his colleague arrived, he examined the lower abdomen and bladder area. His first words were "Your bladder is almost up to your tits!" He quickly went to the nursing desk and called for help.

When the catheter was eventually unplugged, about three quarts (or liters) of urine drained out, much to his relief.

The same surgeon suffered through other instances of poor postoperative treatment, such as inadequate wound care and lack of assistance to move around his room.

Days later, he eventually recovered enough strength to walk unaided, though intravenous lines were still infusing in his left and right arms. He walked to the nursing station and requested a television for his room. The nurse at the station informed him that he had to take his credit card down to the first floor to order a television.

"But that's three floors down and I've got two I.V. poles to lug around." She just stared at him and repeated her statement.

There was no offer of assistance. With credit card in hand, he struggled with his intravenous lines, negotiating the hallways, nooks and crannies of the floors getting into the elevator to go down to the first floor and back to order his television.

"I'm not the type of patient who bugs others for small things. I can't imagine how a non-medical person who has big surgery will get people to look after them. It really scares me," he said.

If a surgeon who understands the system experiences bad care after an operation, imagine the difficulties others might have. His surgery was at a "center of excellence." Yet, there were problems with his postoperative care. There are many mundane yet vitally important procedures that need to be done after surgery; wound care, treating pain and nausea, intravenous fluid infusions, urine output measurements — even simple things like assisting the patient in and out of bed.

Many errors will be made because hospitals are increasingly forced to hire "agency nurses." These are temporary nursing employees who care for patients during nursing shortages. This creates a discontinuity in care, with different people looking after one patient. As well, the quality of care provided by some temporary workers is questionable. Unfortunately, the nursing shortage will only get worse in the future.

How do you ensure good postoperative care? It's important to have a friend or relative follow your recovery on the ward, checking in at least every two to four hours for the first three days. They can inform the nursing desk of problems or complaints, and make sure they're addressed. Because the majority of complications begin in the first 72 hours after surgery, it's essential to have a patient advocate during this period.

CHAPTER 8

Some Cutting Remarks About the Future of the Operating Room

What will the operating room of the future look like? Innovative new devices, instruments and drugs are being introduced all the time. Because so much is happening, many of us struggle to keep informed. Ironically, at the start of our careers, there was a feeling that we had a fairly up-to-date knowledge base. Because we were finally free of those accursed exams, some resolved not to read a single medical article or journal for months. We needed a break.

But as new concepts constantly appear, we realize that keeping up is a lifelong struggle.

Today, the volume of information is overwhelming. A Google search offers millions of references — you've got to be selective when trawling for knowledge. Even after you find what you want, you have to accept that, in many instances, you only have enough time to grasp the basics.

Surgery has undergone huge changes in recent years. In the past, surgeons had to cut and expose large areas of the body in order to visualize and access internal organs. "Exposure, exposure, exposure" was an essential part of technique. Poor, harangued residents would have the scalpel snatched from their hands if they made small incisions in the abdomen. The staff person would then proceed to slash long and deep, while berating the student for not achieving wide exposure.

As mentioned in previous chapters, the trend has shifted towards minimally invasive surgery to avoid large cuts, using long, thin cameras to spy deep into body cavities. Internal organs are manipulated by instruments from outside the body. Ironically, as access to hidden body regions has improved, the surgeon's ability to reach out and directly touch the operated tissue has diminished.

Now, even the way a surgeon performs operations from outside body cavities is changing as is illustrated with robotic surgery. The da Vinci System, made by Intuitive Surgical, allows a surgeon to operate at a distance from the patient while controlling robotic arms that are inserted into body cavities from a remote console.

A high-definition 3-D camera is inserted into the patient and transmits a stereoscopic HD picture to the console screen. Three other robotic arms, called EndoWrists, are also inserted. They're equipped with pincer-type graspers at each end; these cut, grab and cauterize during surgery. They simulate the surgeon's movements at the control console, where small toggle arms with thumb and finger pincer controls are manipulated by the surgeon. Performing the operation requires the skills of a good video gamer.

The toggle pincers scale and dampen the surgeon's tremors and imperfect movements, increasing precision and smoothing motion. Wrist movement by the surgeon is also duplicated by EndoWrists. Surgery performed in confined spaces and awkward angles with these flexible EndoWrists is executed more skillfully than by hand because contracted areas constrain free finger movement. Videos of EndoWrists performing origami attest to the tremendous dexterity operating surgeons possess at the console.

Haptic feedback is another development changing the way surgery will be performed and experienced. The feel and texture of internal organs when touched by remotely controlled instruments will be translated back to cybergloves worn by the surgeon at the remote console. In other words, the toggle controllers simulating the feeling of tissue allow the surgeon to operate as if his hands are inside the body. It helps the surgeon to virtually experience the intimacy of old-time surgery.

Some anesthetics are going to be done robotically and remotely as well. McGill University has developed "McSleepy." This robotic system monitors pain, stress, awareness and muscle relaxation during an operation. An automated computerized system of sensors and feedback loops closely modifies anesthesia drug delivery to keep the patient asleep, stress-free and muscle-relaxed during surgery — in much the same way as auto-pilot can safely fly a plane during long flights.

The robot is definitely faster than the human in adjusting to monitored changes; what robot is momentarily distracted by a telephone call, a good story or daydreams about Angelina Jolie? But seriously, the machine's reactions are instantaneous, and it recalibrates quickly, ready for the next change.

Do I feel threatened by robots performing some of my job? Definitely not. If they can do it safely, and I can supervise via video monitor, it's good for the patient. However, I don't want to end up like some overpaid radiologists, sitting at home by a monitor, sipping tea, examining downloaded images, then dictating, "Some abnormal shadows detected. Suggest follow-up in a few days." Recently, there have been complaints in many hospitals' O.R.s about recently graduated radiologists who are extremely well paid yet unwilling to act conscientiously or cooperatively with others — for example, they are very reluctant to come to the hospital to perform emergency CTs, though they are on call. I just hope the future of the operating room includes more cooperative radiologists.

No matter how technology changes the way we perform surgery, the fundamental factor determining quality and safety of an operation is teamwork. In his book *Complications: A Surgeon's Notes on an Imperfect Science*, writer and surgeon Dr. Atul Gawande argues that surgical teams who work together as partners — discussing and debriefing each other — have the best outcomes when trying to master new techniques.

A paper in the *New England Journal of Medicine* has shown that surgical checklists done before starting operations reduce errors by one-third and deaths by more than 40 percent. A fundamental rule when performing the checklist is that all members of the O.R. team must participate, so each person verifies the others' responsibilities. It helps everyone in the team to watch each other's backs. Again, it demonstrates the value of teamwork.

I recently met a woman who underwent a successful emergency appendectomy. She told me she was not too nervous before surgery — she was actually very confident that everything would work out well. I asked her to explain the reasons for her confidence, to which she replied, "I have a friend who is an O.R. nurse. She said that if all the people looking after you — from nurses in the emergency and operating rooms, to all the doctors who saw you — seemed happy and worked well together, then you're going to be in good hands."

She was absolutely right.

REFERENCES

Chapter 1

Euliano, T. Y., et al. "A Brief Pharmacology Related to Anesthesia." *Essential Anesthesia from Science to Practice*, Cambridge University Press (2004): 173.

MacDonald, A. G., et al. "A Brief Historical Review of Non-Anaesthetic Causes of Fires and Explosions in the Operating Room." *British Journal of Anesthesia*, Vol 73, No 6 (1994): 847–856.

Melling, A. C., et al. "Effects of Preoperative Warming on the Incidence of Wound Infection After Clean Surgery: A Randomized Controlled Trial." *Lancet*, Vol 358 (2001): 876–880.

Sessler, D., et al. "Consequences and Treatment of Perioperative Hypothermia." *Anesthesiology Clinics of North America*, Vol 12 (1994): 425–456.

Chapter 3

Berman, I., et al. "Psychiatrists' Attitudes Toward Psychiatry." *Academic Medicine*, No 71, Issue 2 (1996): 110–111.

Bernardini, M. Q., et al. "Imaging of Lymph Node Metastasis in Cervical Cancer." *Canadian Medical Association Journal,* Vol 178, No 7 (March 25, 2008): 867–869.

Brontel, N., et al. "Seroprevalence of *H. pylori* Infection Among Gastroenterologists in France." *Gut.* No 37 (1995): 310.

Crane, M. "Pop culture: No Fluff, Please, We're Doctors." *Medical Economics,* Vol 77, No 19 (2000): 121–122, 125–127.

Freedman, B. *The Ultimate Guide to Choosing a Medical Specialty,* McGraw-Hill Medical (2007).

Graninetti, D. "Sex and the Satisfied Doctor." *Medical Economics,* Vol 9 (2000): 62.

Hughes, P. H., et al. "Physician Substance Use by Medical Specialty." *Journal of Addictive Diseases,* Vol 18, Issue 2 (1999): 23–37.

Markert, R. J., et al. "Personality as a Prognostic Factor for Specialty Choice." *Medscape Journal of Medicine,* Vol 10, No 2 (2008): 49.

Rollman, B. "Medical Specialty and the Incidence of Divorce." *New England Journal of Medicine,* Vol 336 (March 13, 1997): 800–803.

Wallick, M. M., and K. M. Cambre. "Personality Types in Academic Medicine." *Journal of the Louisiana State Medical Society,* Vol 151 (1999): 378–382.

Zeidow, P. B., et al. "Personality Profiles and Specialty Choices of Students from Two Medical School Classes." *Academic Medicine,* Vol 66, No 5 (May 1991): 283–287.

Chapter 4

Birkmeyer, J. D., et al. "Surgeon Volume and Operative Mortality in the United States," *New England Journal of Medicine,* Vol 349, No 22 (2003): 2117–2127.

Carlin, A. M., et al. "Effect of the 80 Hour Work Week on Resident Operative Experience in General Surgery," *American Journal of Surgery,* Vol 193, No 3 (2007): 326–329.

Chiasson, P., et al. "Minimally Invasive Surgery Training in Canada: A Survey of General Surgery Residents," *Surgical Endoscopy*, Vol 17, No 3 (2003): 371–377.

Chou, B. "Simulators and Virtual Reality in Surgical Education," *Obstetrics and Gynecology Clinics*, Vol 33, No 2 (2006).

Feaning, M. A., et al. "Impact of 80 Hour Work Week on Resident Emergency Operative Experience," *American Journal of Surgery*, Vol 190 (2005): 947–949.

Gawande, A., et al. "Analysis of Errors Reported by Surgeons at Three Teaching Hospitals," *Surgery*, Vol 133, No 6 (2003): 614–621.

Netal, S., et al. "Virtual Reality Training Improves Operating Room Performance," *Annals of Surgery*, Vol 236, No 4 (2002): 458–464.

Rosser, J. C., et al. "The Impact of Video Games on Training Surgeons in the 21st Century," *Archives of Surgery*, Vol 142, No 2 (2007): 181–186.

Rosser, J. C., et al. "Skill Acquisition and Assessment for Laparoscopic Surgery," *Archives of Surgery*, Vol 132 (1997): 200–204.

Tracey, J., et al. "CIHI Survey: Volumes and Outcomes for Surgical Services in Canada," *Healthcare Quarterly*, Vol 8, No 4 (2005): 28–30.

Chapter 5

Roulson, J., et al. "Discrepancies Between Clinical and Autopsy Diagnosis and the Value of Post Mortem Histology: A Meta-Analysis and Review," *Histopathology*, Vol 47, No 6 (2005): 551–559.

Stix, G., "Into the Uncanny Valley," *Scientific American Magazine* (Dec 2008): 24–28.

Chapter 6

Aubrun, F., et al. "Predictive Factors of Severe Postoperative Pain in the Postanesthesia Care Unit," *Anesthesia and Analgesia*, Vol 106 (2008): 1535–1541.

Day Surgery: Development and Practice, International Association for Ambulatory Surgery, Classica Artes Grancas, Porto (2006).

Gan, T. "Risk Factors for Postoperative Nausea and Vomiting," *Anesthesia and Analgesia*, Vol 102 (2006): 1884–1898.

Gandhi, K., et al. "Multimodal Pain Management Techniques in Hip and Knee Arthroplasties," *Journal of New York School of Regional Anesthesia*, Vol 13 (2009).

Janssen, K. J. M., et al. "The Risk of Severe Postoperative Pain: Modification and Validation of a Clinical Prediction Rule," *Anesthesia and Analgesia*, Vol 107 (2008): 1300–1339.

Lavenai, C., et al. "Multimodal Pain Management and Arthrofibrosis in Primary Total Knee Arthroplasties," *Journal of Arthroplasty*, Vol 23, No 2 (2008): 323.

Mauermann, W., et al. "A Comparison of Neuraxial Block Versus General Anesthesia for Elective Total Hip Replacement: A Meta-Analysis," *Anesthesia and Analgesia*, Vol 103 (2006): 1018–1025.

Peter, H., et al. "Post Discharge Nausea and Vomiting and Impact on Functional Quality of Living," *Anesthesia and Analgesia*, Vol 107 (2008): 429–438.

Rathmell, J. P., et al. "The Role of Intrathecal Drugs in the Treatment of Acute Pain," *Anesthesia and Analgesia*, Vol 101 (2005): 530–543.

Scott, S. R., et al. "A Prospective Randomized Trial on the Role of Celecoxib Administration for Total Knee Arthroplasties: Improving Clinical Outcomes," *Anesthesia and Analgesia*, Vol 106 (2008): 1258–1264.

Chapter 7

Amin, A. K., et al. "Total Knee Replacement in Morbidly Obese Patients," *Journal of Bone and Joint Surgery*, Vol 88-B, No 10 (2006): 1321–1326.

Leslie, K., et al. "Dreaming During Anesthesia and Anesthetic Depth in Elective Surgery Patients: A Prospective Cohort Study," *Anesthesiology*, Vol 106 (2007): 33–42.

Malby, J. B. "Preoperative Fasting Guidelines," *Update in Anesthesia*, Vol 12, No 2 (2000): 1–2.

Murphy, R. J., et al. "Homologous Blood Transfusion as a Risk Factor for Postoperative Infection after Coronary Artery Bypass Graft Operations," *Journal of Thoracic and Cardiovascular Surgery*, Vol 124 (1992): 1092–1099.

Nasarway, S., et al. "Morbid Obesity as an Independent Determinant of Death Among Surgical Critically Ill Patients," *Critical Care Medicine*, Vol 34, No 4 (2006): 964–970.

Pescatori, M., et al. "Perioperative Blood Transfusion for the Recurrence of Colorectal Cancer," *Cochrane Database of Systematic Reviews*, No 1 (2006).

Chapter 8

Feder, B. "Prepping Robots to Perform Surgery," *New York Times* (May 4, 2008).

Hayes, A., et al. "A Surgical Safety Checklist to Reduce Morbidity and Mortality in a Global Population," *New England Journal of Medicine*, Vol 360, No 5 (2009): 491–499.

Ubelacker, S., et al. "Canadian Researchers Develop Automated Anesthesia System Dubbed McSleepy," The Canadian Press (May 2, 2008).

ACKNOWLEDGMENTS

I want to thank Jack David, Erin Creasey and the team at ECW Press for their support and assistance. Also, thank you to Loris Lesynski and Dr. Jacqueline Auguste for encouraging me to write this book.